Manuel Lobo

Geographical Distribution of Nurses in Portugal

Manuel Lobo

Geographical Distribution of Nurses in Portugal

Gini Index and OLS Model

ScienciaScripts

Imprint
Any brand names and product names mentioned in this book are subject to trademark, brand or patent protection and are trademarks or registered trademarks of their respective holders. The use of brand names, product names, common names, trade names, product descriptions etc. even without a particular marking in this work is in no way to be construed to mean that such names may be regarded as unrestricted in respect of trademark and brand protection legislation and could thus be used by anyone.

Cover image: www.ingimage.com

This book is a translation from the original published under ISBN 978-613-9-65392-8.

Publisher:
Sciencia Scripts
is a trademark of
Dodo Books Indian Ocean Ltd. and OmniScriptum S.R.L publishing group

120 High Road, East Finchley, London, N2 9ED, United Kingdom
Str. Armeneasca 28/1, office 1, Chisinau MD-2012, Republic of Moldova, Europe
Printed at: see last page
ISBN: 978-620-7-77506-4

GENERAL TABLE OF CONTENTS

SUMMARY

Health services in Portugal are currently facing a number of constraints, both in terms of budget and human resources. It is therefore particularly important that they have an adequate distribution of resources, according to the needs of the population. As far as the distribution of nurses in Portugal is concerned, there is very little literature available in Portugal that looks at and studies the distribution of nurses in Portugal and their respective motivations. For this reason, it was decided to carry out a study to assess the statistics on the distribution of nurses in Portugal at county level and for the years 2002 to 2010, obtained from the National Statistics Institute's database, putting them into context with OECD countries. Variables believed to influence the distribution of the number of nurses in Portugal were taken from the same database. This will be done by evaluating the distribution of the number of nurses at county level using the Gini index, which shows the equity or inequity of the distribution of health professionals. This index showed that there were improvements between 2002 and 2010, but that despite this, there are still inequities in the distribution of nurses in Portugal. After this evaluation, the OLS methodology will also be used, according to the static and dynamic model. The aim of this method is to verify the aspects that influence the distribution of nurses in 2002 and 2010. More than that, the result of the dynamic model will be shown, which aims to demonstrate the factors that seem to have influenced the changes in the growth rates of the distribution of the number of nurses at county level between 2002 and 2010. What emerges is that the number of nurses per thousand inhabitants is positively influenced by variables such as the number of doctors and the number of beds, in line with expectations and the observed literature. What is surprising is the high influence of the purchasing power index on its distribution and the growing influence of eminently demographic variables such as the ageing index and the old-age dependency index.

KEYWORDS: Distribution of nurses, Portugal, Gini index, *OLS* model

INTRODUCTION

The nursing profession has such a long history, with references to the existence of nurses in Portugal dating back to 1120, a date that predates the formation of Portugal by 23 years (Nunes, 2003). Over the course of its existence, changes have been made in line with developments and health needs in Portugal. Important milestones in its evolution include the formation of the National Health System in 1979 (Portal da Saùde, 2011), which led to great progress in terms of both human and material resources in Portugal, and the formation of the Order of Nurses in 1998, which made it possible to regulate the practice of the profession (OE, 2011d). It was precisely after this date that public and private nursing schools began to proliferate, and there are currently 41 of them (DGES, 2012). These have allowed for the continuous growth, development and visibility of nursing professionals (Mendes & Mantovani, 2010).

Given the importance of the nursing profession, its weight in the National Health System and the growing demand for health care, it is important to characterize it and analyse its distribution. In fact, some studies clearly point out the importance of nurses in reducing mortality among patients (Meadows, Levenson & Baeza, 2000 and Aiken, Clarke, Cheung, Sloane & Silber, 2003) and the need to broaden and adapt their functional content so that, in specific contexts, they can contribute to improving healthcare provision (Buchan & Calman, 2005; Marques, 2006; Maynard, 2006).

In this sense, this research project will look at the role of nurses as professionals, as well as their role in the National Health System, with the aim of creating conditions for reflection on the adequacy of their number in relation to health needs and the reasons for their distribution at municipal level in Portugal. The aim of this research is also to reflect on the number of nurses in Portugal in relation to the reality in other developed countries, despite the existence of specific economic, political and social differences between these countries.

International literature describes a general shortage of these professionals (Berlinier & Ginzberg, 2002; Buchan, 2002; Budge, Carryer & Wood, 2003; Tierney, 2003) while there are studies that describe relatively high patterns of demand for health care (Bloor & Maynard, 2003; Birch, O'Brien-Palas, Alksnis, Murphy & Thompson, 2003). Only scattered quantitative statistical data on nursing activity can be found for Portugal, and there is no scientific study on the subject that uses the available statistical information to explain the distribution of nursing professionals across the country's municipalities. To date, there is no known study that has looked into the meaning of these figures, how they fit in with the European reality in particular and the world reality in general, and the factors that influence them. Nor have we had access to guidelines for possible health criteria or policies and the distribution of these professionals throughout the country. Only a study by Correia and Veiga (2009) is known for the Portuguese economy, which describes major disparities in terms of the distribution of doctors at municipal level. These same authors attribute these disparities mainly to inequalities in the distribution of salaries in the different municipalities in Portugal.

Internationally, the studies carried out by Lin, Burns and Nochajski (1997) stand out. These authors show that there is a greater concentration of nurses in urban areas, and that this concentration is positively related to that of doctors and also, but to a lesser extent, to purchasing power. Also, the work of Wong, Watson and Young (2009) reveals that the geographical distribution of primary health care is similar to that of doctors and is not related to the health indices of the population covered by these professionals. As for nurses' motivations for choosing certain regions within countries (more rural or more urban), Skillman, Palazzo, Keepnews and Hart (2005) and Henwood, Eley, Parker, Tucket and Hegney (2009) found that nurses working in rural areas tend to earn lower salaries and work longer hours, due to the smaller supply of nurses, which makes these regions less attractive to these professionals. In addition, according to the same authors, these nurses tend to have lower qualifications than nurses working in urban areas and are more inclined to move to other areas.

In view of the above, the purpose of this work is to describe and analyze the distribution of nurses at the municipal level, analyzing and quantifying their possible motivations. The aim is to go beyond the traditional descriptive quantitative analysis of the number of nurses in Portugal. This will be presented to frame the econometric study and will use statistical information on the national distribution of nurses, provided by the National Institute of Statistics and the Order of Nurses. To make the international comparison, statistical data provided by the Organization for Economic Cooperation and Development (OECD) will be used. To analyze the distribution of nurses by municipality, identify and quantify the factors that influence it, the ordinary least squares econometric methodology will be used (Correia and Veiga, 2010; Lin et al., 1997). The aim of this methodology is to see whether and how a certain set of demographic, economic and healthcare supply variables influence the geographical distribution of nurses. Some of the variables used are: the number of doctors per thousand inhabitants, the number of beds per thousand inhabitants, the existence (or not) of a central hospital, the ageing index, the total population, the old-age dependency index, the masculinity index, the mortality rate and the purchasing power index. These variables were also tested in the studies by Correia and Veiga (2010), Toyabe (2009) and Lin et al. (1997).

Another set of variables was chosen with the aim of verifying whether health, morbidity and population characteristics influence the distribution of nurses in Portugal. It was decided to choose the resident population aged 0 to 14, the ageing index, the longevity index, the masculinity index of people over 65 and the ratio of nurses to doctors. It should be noted that all the variables selected are detailed down to county level.

In addition, the Gini index will be calculated to analyze the equity (or iniquity) of the distribution of these professionals throughout the national territory. This coefficient has been particularly used in the health sector. For example, in the works by Correia and Veiga (2010) and Toyabe (2009) to measure the equity of the geographical distribution of professionals.

In order to achieve the proposed objective, this work will essentially be divided into two chapters.

The first chapter aims to provide a theoretical framework on what the nursing profession is and how it has evolved in Portugal since its inception. It also aims to offer a perspective on the functions and functional content of nurses, in order to understand the specificities of this profession. The chapter will present some literature on the supply of nurses in the healthcare market.

The second chapter is divided into two parts. The first subsection of the second chapter aims to provide a statistical framework for the nursing profession in Portugal and in a selection of OECD countries in their various contexts, while also seeking to compare this reality with the economic and health data from these same countries. In the second subsection, an empirical econometric study is carried out on the distribution of nurses in Portugal, at county level, using the OLS methodology in order to understand which variables influence the distribution of nurses for the years 2002, 2010 and the respective variation between the two periods. The years were selected in order to simultaneously understand the evolution of the distribution of nurses in Portugal over time. In particular, the year 2002 was chosen because it was the first year for which we had all the information we considered relevant at the municipality level. The year 2010 was chosen because it was the last year for which statistical information was available. In addition, the Gini coefficient was calculated to assess the equity of the distribution of these health professionals.

CHAPTER I

NURSING IN PORTUGAL

1.1. A BRIEF HISTORY OF NURSING AND ITS EVOLUTION TO THE PRESENT DAY

According to Rosado, Rolo, Silva and Castel-Branco (2007, p.7), the practice of nursing is as "old as the very existence of man". According to Robinson (1946), women are born instinctive nurses, naturally providing care to all those who need it. Donahue (1996) also believes that women are considered nurses from birth due to their "maternal instinct", to which scientific knowledge, skill and specialization have been added.

The role of nurses began with caring for sick, elderly, disabled and terminally ill people, and has evolved over time. In Portugal, there are references to the existence of nurses as far back as 1120, a date that predates the formation of the country itself by 23 years. At that time, reports from other parts of the world indicated that care for the sick and infirm was provided by monks and nuns (Nunes, 2003).

Despite the long-standing accounts of health care providers, the origins of modern nursing really came about, according to Rosado et al. (2007), with the teachings of Florence Nightingale (1820-1910) who, having come into contact with various episodes of war, quickly joined various religious orders that cared for the wounded. In this environment, she took the first steps towards making nursing more scientific, distancing herself from the empirical and religious care of the time. Proof of this was the emphasis he placed on the systematic collection of statistical data, which served as the basis for the first research work in the field. The exponent of her publications was *Notes on Nursing* (Nightingale, 1860), in which she pointed to drinking water, ventilation, room hygiene and basic sanitation (just to name a few examples) as important factors in maintaining the health of her patients. Until then, these factors were completely ignored by healthcare providers. This innovative spirit, the "environmental model" she created (Nightingale, 1860) and pioneering research theories mean that Florence Nightingale is considered the patron saint of modern nursing. Thus, an important milestone in the history of nursing took place in 1860, with the opening of the first nursing school, the *Nightingale School of Nurses* (Rosado et al., 2007).

In Portugal, the first known act relating to nursing education came from Costa Simões who, in 1881, implemented the first course for nurses at the Coimbra University Hospitals. Although the course was not particularly successful, it contributed to the fact that, on December 9, 1885, Tomâs de Carvalho, head nurse of the Hospital Real Sâo José, asked the government for authorization to open the first nursing school, under the pretext of the need to contain costs. This came to fruition in January 1886 (Rosado et al., 2007 and Graça & Henriques, 2000).

However, according to Nogueira (1990), the first professional nursing school was only founded in 1901 at the S. José Hospital, where the course lasted two years. Its aim was to train professionals capable of enforcing medical prescriptions and thus contributing to better treatment for patients. From this time onwards, nursing schools proliferated and, consequently, the number of nurses has grown to the present day. The technical and organizational aspects of the profession have become increasingly sophisticated as a result of the improvement in the quality and conditions of teaching. It should be noted that there is currently a wide range of nursing schools - there are 41 nursing schools in Portugal, of which 20 are private and 21 are public (DGES, 2012).

Despite their growing importance in the provision of health care, it wasn't until 1981 that the Nursing Career Diploma was published by Decree-Law No. 305/81 of November 12, which enshrined nurses in a single career. This law also defined the various nursing categories, from the lowest grade (nursing technician) to the highest (nurse supervisor and head nurse)[1] . In 1983, nursing specialties were created, such as obstetrics, rehabilitation, public health, mental and psychiatric health and child and pediatric health (Quintas, Farto, Rosa & Santos, 2007). In the 1990s, two more landmark events took place: The first was the creation of the Order of Nurses (OE), with the approval of its statutes in Decree-Law No. 104/98 of April 21 (1998). In this way, the profession took important steps towards its effective consolidation and towards improving the regulation of professional practice. Another important event took place in 1999 with the integration of the Nursing Schools into higher education, namely with the awarding of the academic degree of licenciatura to the nursing course by Decree-Law No. 353/99 of September 3 (Nunes, 2003).

From 2000 to the present day, the Ordem dos Enfermeiros (Order of Nurses) has asserted itself as the entity that regulates the practice of Portuguese nursing. In particular, the creation of quality standards in nursing, with the aim of regularizing and standardizing the quality standards of nursing practice (OE, 2011a).

1.2. FRAMEWORK FOR NURSING IN THE PORTUGUESE NATIONAL HEALTH SERVICE

The development of the nursing profession has evolved in tandem with the progress and

1 This subject will be covered in more detail in the following chapters.

evolution of the health system in Portugal. It is therefore important to understand how the health system has evolved in Portugal and how some health indicators have evolved. According to Bentes, Dias, Sakellarides and Bankauskaite (2004), the health system in Portugal, before the 18th century, was limited to hospitals and religious institutions, called Misericórdias, which essentially provided support to the poor and disadvantaged. In the 18th century, the kingdom began to establish a very limited number of public hospitals, mainly university hospitals, so that students (mainly doctors) could practice and thus provide some support to the community. The public health service itself only began in 1901, when the first legislation was passed creating a national network of doctors to help the population (Bentes et al., 2004). Since then, it wasn't until 1946 that there was a paradigm shift due to the ideologies introduced by German Bismack, whose model argued that health should cover the employed population and their dependents and be financed by social security and sickness funds. This model of compulsory contributions[2] gave rise to the Welfare Fund Federation and would continue into the 1970s (Portal da Saùde, 2011).

According to Baganha, Ribeiro and Pires (2002), at the end of the 1960s, the only health institutions in existence were Misericórdias and centuries-old social solidarity institutions, essentially located in large urban centers. There was also the possibility of resorting to private services, only available to higher social strata. According to Bentes et al. (2004) these facts were compounded by various socio-cultural problems such as the asymmetrical distribution of health care, unhealthy sanitary conditions and the lack of coordination between the different health institutions[3] . Of course, all these situations had their consequences for the health of the Portuguese population, such as a high infant mortality rate[4] as we'll see below.

Looking at some statistics provided by the Organization for Economic Cooperation and Development (OECD)[5] , it can be seen that public health care was not at the top of the priorities of the Portuguese governments of the time. Public spending on health, as a percentage of Gross Domestic Product (GDP), was only 2.4% in 1970. This figure was the lowest of the OECD countries, a far cry from countries like Canada, the United States of America (USA) and Denmark, which allocated 7.2%, 7.3% and 7.9% of GDP, respectively,

---

2 A compulsory contribution is understood as a worker giving up part of his or her salary so that it can be used for the common good (Ricardo, 1965).

3 Due to the fact that power was centralized (we lived in a dictatorial political regime in a country with few means of communication).

4 Throughout this research paper, various statistical data will be presented that describe the reality of health indicators in Portugal over time.

5 OECD Health Statistics database: http://stats.OCDE.org/Index.aspx?DataSetCode=HEALTH_STAT.

to health care spending. It should be noted that the amount spent on health *per capita* by the state was the lowest in the OECD (47 US dollars), while the highest was in the US with 311 US dollars *per capita*. This is all the more significant given that the average amount spent on health in OECD countries at that time was 196 dollars. The fact is that there is no consensus in the literature consulted and reviewed about the right percentage of GDP to use to produce better health indicators. For Richardson (1997), in principle, the ideal GDP resources to allocate to health should depend on the extent to which the expected health benefits outweigh the costs. A study by Briggs, King, Basu and Stuckler (2010) revealed that increases in GDP have a considerably positive impact on the health of the population, so the strength of the relationship is strongly influenced by changes in levels of poverty and inequality, which are generally attenuated in growing economies. In other words, growing economies have citizens with a better state of health, because the state has the capital to invest more in health and citizens have greater purchasing power. Also noteworthy are the potential years of life lost[6] per 100,000 people in the Portuguese population at the time. In 1970, these were among the highest in the OECD, with 11,810.5 potential years of life lost per 100,000 inhabitants for women and 17,404.1 for men. Countries such as Iceland, Norway and the Netherlands had lower figures[7] at around 5,061, 5,220 and 5,238 potential years of life lost per 100,000 inhabitants, respectively (OECD, 2011a). These figures clearly indicated deficiencies in the health system at the time, as people were dying earlier than expected.

However, according to Baganha et al. (2002), some signs of change began to appear at the beginning of the 1970s, namely with the introduction of Decree-Law No. 413/71 of 27 September (1971), which recognized the right to health for all citizens. It was also through this legal regulation and Decree-Law No. 414/71 of 27 September that the so-called Ministry of Health and Assistance was completely organized. In this way, the state became responsible for both health policy and its implementation and promotion (Portal da Saùde, 2011). With these foundations laid, 1979 saw the birth of the National Health System [SNS] through Decree-Law 56/79 of September 15. Under this law, access to healthcare is guaranteed to all citizens, regardless of their economic and social status (Portal da Saùde, 2011). Associated with these transformations in Portuguese society, the 1970s saw, according to Barros (1999), the beginning of the biggest reforms in the Portuguese health system, in that serious progress was made due essentially to an increase in investment in

6 The number of years that a given population will theoretically stop living if they die prematurely (before the age of 70) (OECD, 2000).

7 It should be understood that, in this case, lower values of potential years of life lost represent better results, as it means that people live more years in relation to their life expectancy.

health. This investment was essentially in facilities (hospitals and health centers) and in improving the training and number of health professionals (doctors, nurses and health technicians) (Pinto & Aragâo, 2003).

Having briefly presented the historical background and the institutional context in which the nursing professional operates, it is important to describe what a nurse does. As they cover a wide area, we will present their essential competencies and the functional content of their activity.

1.3. COMPETENCIES AND FUNCTIONAL CONTENT OF THE NURSING PROFESSION

Over the last few years, nursing has evolved considerably, both in terms of its basic training and in terms of the complexity and dignity of its professional practice (OE, 2011b).

A nurse is a professional with a legally recognized nursing degree who has been awarded a professional title that recognizes scientific, technical and human competence to provide nursing care to individuals (OE, 2011c). According to Decree-Law no. 161/96, of September 4 (p. 2960), nursing is the profession that aims to "provide nursing care to healthy or sick human beings, so that they can maintain, improve and recover their health, helping them to reach their maximum functional capacity as quickly as possible".

Given the development and proliferation of the profession, it was necessary to create appropriate legislation to regulate its practice. Decree-Law no. 161/96 of September 4 was therefore approved in 1996, regulating the practice of nursing in Portugal. This decree-law was repealed by Decree-Law No. 104/98 of April 21 (1998), due to the creation of the Order of Nurses, which now had legal and autonomous instruments to regulate the profession. As such, by imposition of Decree-Law No. 104/98, the practice of nursing became conditional on obtaining a professional card, issued by the Order of Nurses (OE, 2011d). This regulation of the profession was intended to meet Portuguese society's expectations of this professional group (OE, 2011b). As such, it was only since then that the number of nurses in Portugal began to be properly controlled and monitored, which is reflected in the amount of statistical data that has come into existence since then and which will be analyzed later in this paper. Table 1 shows the number of nurses registered with the Order of Nurses in Portugal since 2000 and who are active (working). The table also differentiates between specialist and generalist (non-specialist) nurses. The figures are up to 2010, the last year for which data is available.

Table 1

Distribution of generalist and specialist nurses in Portugal from 2000 to 2010

Specialty	Year										
	2000	2001	2002	2003	2004	2005	2006	2007	2008	2009	2010
General Nurse	30.883	32.855	35.112	37.182	39.172	41.440	44.069	46.443	48.401	50.040	51.903
Specialist Nurse	6.740	6.794	6.790	6.796	6.734	6.856	7.032	7.785	8.465	9.715	10.673
Total	37.623	39.649	41.902	43.978	45.906	48.296	51.101	54.228	56.866	59.755	62.566
Annual growth rate (%)		5,39	5,68	4,95	4,38	5,21	5,81	6,12	4,86	5,08	4,70
Average growth rate 2000-2010 (%)						5,22					

Source: Adapted from Ordem dos Enfermeiros: statistical data 2000-2010 (OE, 2011f)

As can be seen, from 2000 to 2010, the growth in the total number of nurses has been consistent, with annual growth rates of between 4 and 6%. The average growth rate between 2000 and 2010 was 5.22%, which confirms the upward trend seen in the absolute numbers. This increase has not been unrelated to the increase in the number of schools (DGES, 2012) and the growing appreciation and visibility of the nursing profession (Mendes & Mantovani, 2010).

The nursing career, previously approved by Decree-Law 437/91 of November 8, had five categories: nurse, graduate nurse, specialist nurse, head nurse and nurse supervisor. This system was recently amended by Decree-Law No. 248/2009 of September 22 and Decree-Law No. 122/2010 of November 11, essentially with the aim of providing remuneration that is more in line with the increasing degree of functional and training complexity of the nursing profession (OE, 2011e).

In terms of nursing specialties, according to the OE (2011e), there are postgraduate specialization courses in nursing: community nursing, medical-cirurgical nursing, rehabilitation nursing, child health/pediatric nursing, maternal health/obstetric nursing and, finally, mental health/psychiatric nursing, as can be seen in Table 2. This table shows the number of nurses distributed among the different specialties between 2000 and 2010.

Table 2

Distribution of nurses by specialty in Portugal from 2000 to 2010

Specialty	Year										
	2000	2001	2002	2003	2004	2005	2006	2007	2008	2009	2010
Rehabilitation	1.017	1.023	1.027	1.033	1.029	1.049	1.111	1.233	1.403	1.745	1.962
Child Health	961	973	978	982	989	987	1.044	1.196	1.314	1.498	1.649
Maternal Health	1.576	1.576	1.556	1.553	1.516	1.641	1.699	1.898	2.032	2.174	2.329
Public Health	584	576	563	-	-	-	-	-	-	-	-

Medico-Cirurgical	1.141	1.157	1.175	1.177	1.176	1.179	1.194	1.275	1.365	1.578	1.767
Community Health	478	500	513	1.082	1.076	1.069	1.078	1.247	1.349	1.545	1.699
Mental Health	983	989	978	969	948	931	906	936	1.002	1.173	1.264
Total	6.740	6.794	6.790	6.796	6.734	6.856	7.032	7.785	8.465	9.715	10.673
Annual growth rate (%)		0,80	-0,06	0,09	-0,91	1,81	2,57	10,71	8,73	14,77	9,86
Average growth rate 2000-2010 (%)						4,70					

Source: Own elaboration based on data from Ordem dos Enfermeiros: statistical data 2000-2010 (OE, 2011f).

As can be seen, the total number of specialist nurses has shown a general upward trend from 2000 to 2010 (4.7% on average per year). The exceptions are 2002 and 2004, when the total number of specialist nurses showed negative annual growth rates. In 2010, the most popular specialties were maternal health and rehabilitation, and the least popular was mental health. It should be noted that from 2003 there was no longer a public health nursing specialty, since its functional content was overlapping with other health technicians (environmental health technicians) trained for this purpose since 1993 (Graça & Henriques, 2000). Public health nurses moved to the community health specialty[8] , which explains the large increase in the number of nurses in this specialty between 2002 and 2003.

With regard to the different specialties of the nursing profession, the following should be mentioned in order to gain a better understanding of the activity carried out. Rehabilitation nursing plays an important role in improving the quality of life and independence of the individual[9] , as the nurse goes into the home to rehabilitate patients who are usually totally dependent. The medical-surgical, mental health (psychiatry), child health (paediatrics) and maternal health (obstetrics) specialties are aimed at the development and continuous specialization of nurses in their specific fields, allowing them to obtain skills that will enable them to *perform* better in more complex and specific areas of their daily lives. These specializations enable better personal preparation, allowing access to better pay and more differentiated and autonomous positions (ESENFC, 2011). On this subject, it is interesting to note that, according to Buchan and Calman (2005), surveys carried out on users of healthcare institutions in the USA and the UK in 2000 show that they are more satisfied with routine consultations with specialist nurses than with clinicians, since the former have

8 The designation of community nursing was the result of a choice made by the competent bodies of the OE, based on Ordinance No. 239/94 of April 16 and the conceptual evolution that has taken place internationally.
9 The text refers, above all, to bedridden patients, at home, who do not have the physical, financial or family support to travel to health institutions for treatment.

more time and more availability for users. Also, in the view of Delamaire and Lafortune (2010), specialist nurses can play a very important role in improving access to health care in the face of a shortage of clinicians, especially in routine follow-ups in primary health care. [10]The authors point out that while countries such as the USA, the UK and Canada have had these routines in place since 1960, this is not the case in other countries, including Portugal. In fact, according to Maynard (2006), in Australia, in order to deal with the lack of clinicians in remote areas, some of the basic tasks of doctors are divided up and delegated to nurses and other health technicians who have the autonomy to diagnose and prescribe a specific range of situations as long as they have the preparation/training to do so and follow the pre-established protocols previously discussed between the different professionals.

Following on from this subject, we will look at the practice of nursing from a more psychological point of view, highlighting the importance of the nursing professional's autonomy in the performance of their profession.

1.3.1. NURSES: ETHICS AND THE IMPORTANCE OF THEIR AUTONOMY

The aim of this subsection is to explain the main premises and rules of conduct for nurses, as well as the importance of their autonomy and actions in promoting the health of patients. According to the code of ethics for nurses[11] , their actions must take into account the concern to defend the dignity of the human person. Their activity must be guided by competence and professional development and have as its guiding principles: (1) the responsibility inherent in the role assumed before society, (2) respect for human rights in the relationship with users and, (3) excellence in the exercise of the profession, in general, and in the relationship with other professionals, in particular. According to Wade (1999, p. 310) nurses' autonomy is an essential attribute and is defined as "conscious and responsible decision-making that reflects the best interests of the patient". The author also lists the following as critical attributes for success: the establishment of an affectionate relationship with the patient, proactive decision-making and interdependence between colleagues.

According to the Nursing Council [CE] of the Order of Nurses, the nurse's focus should always be on the patient, since they are the reason for their existence as a professional. As such, nurses must conduct themselves impartially, providing care regardless of moral, religious or social issues (CE, 2003). In addition, although nurses act in an autonomous,

10 This is reflected in higher current nurse/doctor ratios, as will be seen below.

11 This code is included in the OE Statute, in accordance with Decree-Law 111/2009 of September 16th.

independent and responsible manner, they must not forget that they are part of multidisciplinary teams and are obliged to interact with them, creating synergies and thus bringing benefits to the patient (OE, 2011c). These premises are essential for training good professionals and can make the difference between the life and death of a patient during their professional practice. Aiken (1994) found that in hospitals that were referenced as having good nursing practices, mortality was lower when compared to other hospitals. In other words, a hospital that has a well-prepared, accredited nursing team and conducts itself appropriately can make the difference between life and death. Several studies, such as those by Meadows et al. (2000) and Aiken et al. (2003), have found a relationship between high nurse ratios, better health parameters, reduced risk of complications for patients and reduced hospital mortality. However, despite the fact that better health indices are found in countries with higher public spending on health and a higher concentration of nurses, Simoens (2005) found that it is unclear whether it is the number of nurses that influences spending or spending that influences the number of nurses, since there is no proven correlation between these aspects.

For Carrie, Harvey, West, Mckenna and Keeney (2005), the quality of care provided, the level of education of the nursing team, *the skill-mix*[12] and the autonomy of the nurses are considered essential premises for good nurse conduct, although the study by these authors found no statistical evidence of an association between the four variables. This was not the case with Needelman, Buerhaus, Mattke, Stewart and Zelevinsky (2002, p.1720) who mention the existence of "consistent evidence of an association between higher levels of nurse training and lower rates of adverse effects in users".

Although nurses always have a certain degree of autonomy, they are almost always dependent on doctors for the administration of certain therapies. In fact, according to Lin et al. (1997), the development of nurses has always gone hand in hand with that of doctors, since a significant part of nurses' work is carried out on medical advice/supervision, whether direct or indirect. Studies by Budge et al. (2003) show that the doctor-nurse relationship is essential for improving autonomy, control and quality in the provision of health care.

For Wade (1999), the elements that support the development of nurses' autonomy are continuous training, understanding the work environment and clinical decision-making.

12 According to Cahill (1995) and Marques (2006), the *skill-mix* or "sharing of tasks between professions" is defined as the proportion of staff qualifications in terms of competence, skill, knowledge and experience that are needed to reach a satisfactory standard to meet a given level of demand for health care It was decided to use the original (English) expression in this research work because it is the one that is universally known and used.

Actions carried out by nurses under their sole and exclusive initiative and responsibility are considered autonomous, whether in the provision of care, management, teaching, training or, possibly, nursing research. Autonomy, also known in international terminology as *shared governance*[13] , has, according to Porter (1992), Gavin and Wakefield (1999) and Doherty and Hope (2000), been shown to bring benefits such as increased retention of health professionals, increased morale in the work group, increased participation in decision-making, improved quality and simplification of multidisciplinary work.

According to the *Health at a Glance* report by the OECD (OECD, 2011b), nurses play an increasingly important role in the different health systems. Not only do they provide health care in the traditional hospital sector, but also in long-term care facilities, primary health care and home care, where they are beginning to emerge in force, as mentioned earlier in this paper. In the field of disease prevention, we highlight the work of community nursing, which operates in schools through health prevention and promotion programs, such as the prevention of obesity, respiratory diseases and raising awareness among young people of healthy habits (DGS, 2011).

1.4. HEALTH AND NURSING STATISTICS - PORTUGUESE SITUATION IN THE OECD CONTEXT

As seen above (see Table 1), and according to the Ordem dos Enfermeiros statistical bulletin (OE, 2011f), between 2000 and 2010 the number of nurses registered with the Order grew from 37,487 to 52,566[14] . Figure 1 shows the number of nurses per 1,000 inhabitants in OECD countries in 2000, 2004 and 2008. The selection of these 3 years gives an idea of the quantitative evolution of the number of nurses in the selected countries.

13 *Shared governance* is defined as an "organizational process that legitimizes nurses' control over their practice and extends their influence into some areas that may have previously been controlled by management" (Hess, 1994, p. 28).

14 It should be noted that this is the number of active and effective nurses registered with the Order of Nurses, and not the total number of registered nurses. Throughout the paper, the number of practicing or employed nurses will be used. Finally, it should be noted that in Portugal there is only statistical information on these professionals from 1999 onwards, due to the fact that the OE was only formed in 1998, as has already been mentioned.

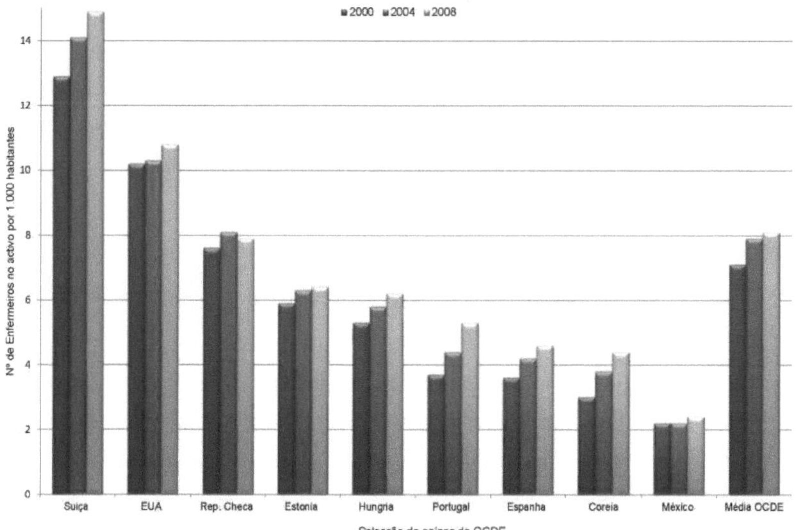

Notes: The statistical data presented refer to the number of active nurses, providing direct care to users, however, for Portugal and Greece the data refer to the number of active nurses, including those in the research and teaching areas.

Figura 1. Number of nurses per 1,000 inhabitants in a group of OECD countries in 2000, 2004 and 2008.

Source: Own elaboration based on *OECD Health Data* [15]

Figure 1 shows an upward trend in the number of nurses per 1,000 inhabitants in all countries, and Portugal is no exception, rising from 3.7 in 2000 to 5.3 in 2008, an increase of around 30%. Despite this upward trend in the number of nurses, the number is still well below the average for OECD countries, which was around 8.1 nurses per 1,000 inhabitants in 2008. For example, the number of nurses per thousand inhabitants in Portugal in 2008 was still below countries like Estonia, Hungary and the Czech Republic. It should be noted that although the USA has one of the highest numbers of nurses per 1,000 inhabitants (10.8), this number is still not considered sufficient to combat the shortage of nurses in this country, as reported by Berlinier and Ginzberg (2002). There was an estimated 12% shortage of nurses in the USA in 2010 (BHP, 2002).

The shortage of nurses is not exclusive to the US. It is estimated that in 2020, there will be a shortage of nearly one million nurses around the world, with the actual number not

15 OECD Health Statistics database: http://stats.OCDE.org/Index.aspx?DataSetCode=HEALTH_STAT.

enough to meet all the needs (Aiken & Cheung, 2008). In fact, several authors such as Berlinier and Ginzberg (2002), Buchan (2002), Budge et al. (2003) and Tierney (2003) state that the shortage of nurses is already a global reality. The ageing of nurses, together with the inversion of the age pyramids[16] , are serious factors of concern for the future (Baumann, Blythe, Kolotylo & Underwood, 2004). This situation has led to a decrease in the ratio of nurses to patients, a situation which, according to Aiken, Clarke, Sloane, Sochalsky and Silber (2002), is clearly harmful as it increases the likelihood of death among patients, the dissatisfaction of the nurses themselves and situations of *Burnout*[17] among these professionals.

It should be noted that, according to Buchan (2002), the problem of a shortage of nurses doesn't just affect them, but the entire health system. This author stresses the need for a thorough review of health policies so that services and their respective professionals are distributed in such a way as to better serve the needs of the population. For Berlinier and Ginzberg (2002, p. 2742), it has become a "commonplace" to note that nurses usually "love their work but hate their jobs". This state of mind reveals that there are deficiencies in hospital hierarchical structures that lead to professional discontent, with negative consequences for their work. It is therefore crucial for team leaders and hospital managers to have a broad perspective on the problems and to be able to resist the pressures of the hospital system, for example by having the courage to change routines, fight against the inertia of the hospital system and vested corporate interests, with the aim of increasing the satisfaction of users, professionals and employers (Buchan, 2002).

In this context, the nurse/doctor ratio is extremely important as it provides a picture of the number of doctors and nurses and their proportion. Furthermore, according to Bigbee (2008), the nurse/doctor ratio seems to be closely related to healthier communities. The higher this ratio, the better the health indices of the country in question[18] . In view of the above, the values for the nurse/doctor ratio in 2009 for some of the different countries that make up the OECD are shown in the following figure (Figure 2).

16 This leads to an increase in demand for health care.

17 According to França (1987), a Burnout situation is characterized by the physical, psychological and emotional exhaustion of an individual, resulting from stressful and excessive work. It is a clinical condition resulting from people's poor adaptation to their work.

18 It should be noted that, although this is an issue of enormous importance and controversy, it will not be analyzed in this work.

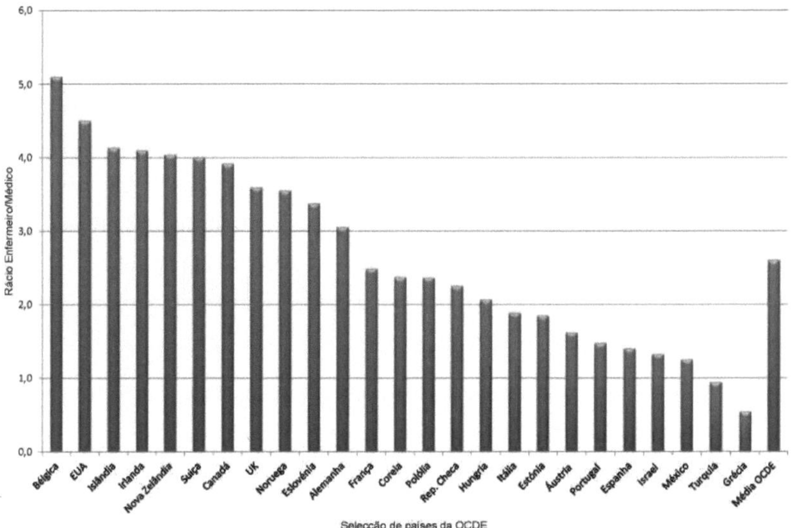

Figura 2. Ratio of nurses to doctors in a selection[19] of OECD countries in 2009.

Source: Own elaboration based on *OECD Health Data*[20]

Looking at the ratio of nurses to doctors, it can be seen that Portugal, with a ratio of 1.5 nurses for every doctor in 2009, is a long way from the average observed for all the OECD countries under analysis, which is 2.6. It is interesting to note that Northern European countries (such as Ireland, Finland and Denmark) have the highest ratios while Mediterranean European countries (such as Greece, Italy, Spain and Portugal) have the lowest ratios.

This ratio, closely related to *skill-mix,* can involve a variety of adaptations such as increasing the skills and responsibilities of a particular group of professionals, in this case between doctors and nurses. In the Northern European countries mentioned above, nurses have more autonomy and there are also good health indicators in these countries (OECD, 2011b). The adaptations mentioned above can be motivated by human resource constraints. For example, in a given service, given the shortage of clinicians, it may be necessary to delegate certain skills to the available professionals, in order to provide greater and better services, boosting capacities (Marques, 2006; Maynard, 2006 and Munga & Maestad, 2009). This aspect is also described by Buchan and Calman (2005),

19 It was decided to use only those countries for which 2009 data on the number of doctors and nurses was available. The average shown is the average of the countries for which data was available - those shown in Figure 2.
20 Health Statistics database: http://stats.OECD.org/Index.aspx?DataSetCode=HEALTH_STAT.

who point out that the readaptation of the *skill-mix* can be due to the scarcity of resources in particular areas (such as inland or rural towns) or by pressures to contain costs and maintain the same health services. Although the *skill-mix* is seen by some authors, such as Gibbs, Mccaughan and Grifits (1991, p. 242) as "highly limiting" and Mckeown (1994, p. 38) as "an explicit attack on the health system". 38) as "an explicit attack on the values of nursing", it is also believed that it increases the level of professionalism of nurses and reduces the incidence of adverse effects to the extent that existing human resources are leveraged and adapted to the needs of certain populations (Carr-Hill & Jenkins-Clarke, 2003; Blegen, Goode & Reed, 1998; Friesen, 1996).

After focusing on all these particular aspects of the nursing profession and activity, as well as a brief statistical framework, the following sections will look at the "market" in which nurses operate and what can influence it.

1.5. SUPPLY AND DEMAND FOR HEALTHCARE IN PORTUGAL

The health market today is very different from traditional markets, not least because of the existence of externalities[21] , uncertainty[22] about the need for health care and the existence of imperfect information between the players. These are all important factors to consider and which condition the market. Unlike other traditional markets, healthcare is a consumer good that does not provide utility on its own. As such, we are dealing with a good that has no intrinsic utility and whose consumption will always be related to a state of need on the part of the demand agent (Matias, 1995). Therefore, before we begin to address this issue, it is important to clarify that the demand for healthcare is different from the need for healthcare (Williams, 1978). That's why, throughout this work, when we refer to demand for healthcare, we mean demand for healthcare, regardless of whether or not there is a need for it. The supply of health care refers to the set of human and material resources available to the population so that they can be provided with adequate health care. Health care is understood as goods or services whose consumption provides health, the latter being a desired state when consuming that good (Matias, 1995). In this sense, the following describes the supply of health care in Portugal in terms of its material and human resources.

21 Externalities are activities that involve the involuntary imposition of costs or benefits (negative or positive) on third parties, without them having the opportunity to prevent it (Barros, 2009).

22 It is defined as a state of uncertainty on the part of patients as to when they will need health care. It can occur between doctor-dentist, patient-insurer, etc. (Barros, 2009).

1.5.1 - HEALTH CARE PROVISION IN PORTUGAL: HUMAN AND MATERIAL RESOURCES[23]

As has already been described, 1971 saw the creation of a health service accessible to all. The first health centers were created, with the aim of providing health care more closely[24] (Branco & Ramos, 2001). In 1974, the first district hospitals and other local health units were created, many of which had previously been owned by the Santa Casa da Misericórdia and were acquired by the state (Bentes et al., 2004). In this way, the distributive map of healthcare provision in Portugal was drawn, culminating in 2009 with the distribution illustrated in Figure 3.

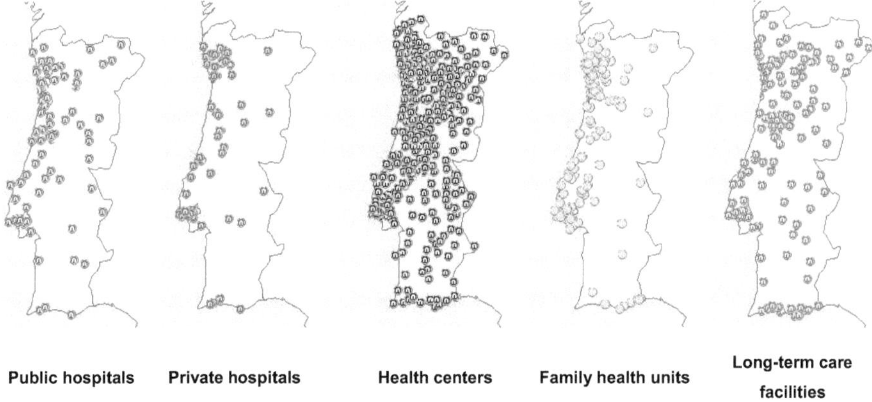

Figure 3 - Distribution map of the network of health institutions in mainland Portugal in 2009

Source: High Commission for Health [ACS] (http://www.websig.acs.min-saude.pt/)

As you can see, there was a greater agglomeration of public and private hospitals in the coastal regions in 2009. The same is true of family health units, which were created more recently, but still seem to be more concentrated in the more populated areas. The situation is different for health centers and long-term care facilities, which are distributed a little more widely throughout Portugal, perhaps due to their original purpose: to provide local health care (Branco & Ramos, 2001).

As for the professionals, their distribution by ACES does not seem to follow any specific pattern, as can be seen in Figure 4.

---

23 In order to check the main indices of existing healthcare provision, we used the High Commission for Health's interactive "Websig" platform, available at http://www.websig.acs.min-saude.pt/.

24 Its activity was essentially centered on the prevention of infectious diseases through vaccination campaigns and assistance to the most vulnerable groups, among other preventive activities (Branco & Ramos, 2001).

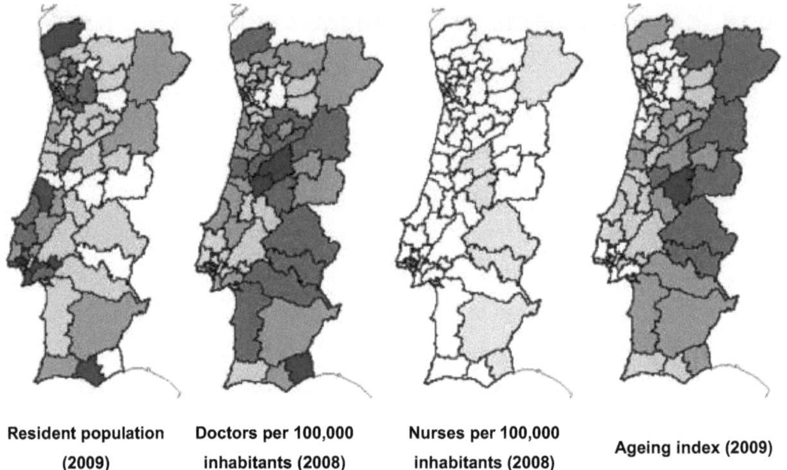

Figure 4 - Distribution of resident population, family doctors, nurses and ageing index, by ACES, in mainland Portugal[25]

Source: High Commission for Health [ACS] (http://www.websig.acs.min-saude.pt/)

As can be seen, the resident population in 2009 in mainland Portugal is particularly concentrated in the coastal regions. With regard to the concentration of doctors, there is a high concentration of family doctors per thousand inhabitants in the ACES of Algarve III[26] and Pinhal Interior Norte I[27] and II[28] . On the other hand, the distribution of the number of nurses per thousand inhabitants does not seem to follow any specific pattern. The distribution of these last professionals shows approximately the same density in Portugal in 2009, although some inland areas show higher numbers of nurses per 100,000 inhabitants. This fact may cause some surprise since, as mentioned in previous sections, the work of nurses is somewhat dependent on medical supervision (Lin et al., 1997; Budge et al., 2003), so it could be assumed that in terms of distribution they could also be "on par". It should also be noted that the ageing index[29] is distributed in the opposite way to the concentration of hospitals and the distribution of the resident population, which shows that inland areas are inhabited especially by older people - traditionally more in need of

25 The analysis refers only to mainland Portugal, as the source consulted does not have data for the Azores and Madeira archipelagos.
26 Agrupamento de Centros de Saùde, Algarve III: includes the municipalities of Castro Marim, Vila Real de Santo Antonio and Tavira (ARS-AL, 2011).
27 Agrupamento de Centros de Saùde Pinhal Interior I: includes the municipalities of Arganil, Gois, Tabua, Oliveira do Hospital, Pampilhosa da Serra, Lousâ, Vila Nova de Poiares and Miranda do Corvo;
28 Agrupamento de Centros de Saùde Pinhal Interior II: includes the municipalities of Figuero dos Vinhos, Penela, Ansiâo, Castanheira de Pera and Alvaiazere (ARS-C, 2011).
29 Obtained from the ratio between the resident population aged over 65 and the resident population aged under 14 (ACS, 2011).

health care. In other words, older people prevail in the inland regions while the distribution of hospitals and the resident population prevails in the coastal regions (ACS, 2011). Ciutan and Chirac (2009) state that a distribution of the number of hospitals based essentially on population criteria (as seems to be the case in Portugal) may not be sufficient to describe the usefulness of that hospital, so hospital network distribution policies should take into account not only quantitative criteria (population covered) but also qualitative criteria (population needs). After describing some data on the supply of healthcare, attention will now be paid to the demand side.

1.5.2 - DEMAND FOR HEALTH CARE IN PORTUGAL

According to the latest censuses carried out in Portugal (in 2010), Portugal has 10,555,853 residents (INE, 2011), 1,700,000 of whom are mainly located in Greater Lisbon and most of whom do not have a family doctor (Mota, 2011). In 2009, the number of medical consultations per inhabitant was 4.5, which corresponds to approximately 47,500,000 million consultations[30] per year. It should be noted that the ratio between hospital emergencies and outpatient consultations is 0.5. This figure indicates that people go to emergency appointments twice as often as they go to scheduled appointments (ACS, 2011). The utilization rate[31] is high in most ACES, as can be seen in the following figure (Figure 5).

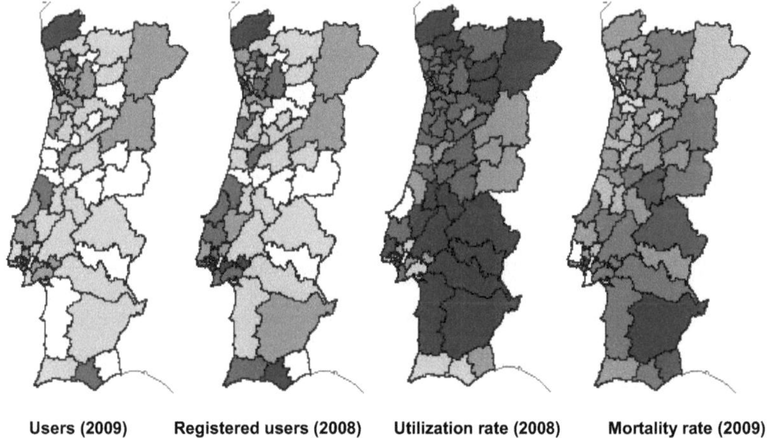

Figura 5. Number of users and registered users, utilization rate and mortality rate, by health

30 This includes consultations at health centers and hospitals.

31 Obtained from the ratio between the number of users with at least one contact with the ACES in a year and the number of users registered with the ACES in the same year (ACS, 2011).

center groupings in mainland Portugal.

Source: High Commission for Health [ACS] (http://www.websig.acs.min-saude.pt/)

Figure 5 shows that there are many similarities between the distribution of registered users and user users (with the exception of the Greater Lisbon region). The utilization rate is high for most ACES. Those with the highest utilization rates are the ACES in the Trás-os-Montes, Minho and Alentejo regions, with figures above 70% in 2008 (ACS, 2011). A utilization rate of this magnitude means that 70% of the population of the ACES had at least one contact with a health institution during 2008, which is quite significant.

It should be noted that although these figures may seem considerable, this influx does not translate into a high number of hospitalizations and discharges[32] , according to the *Health at a Glance* report issued by the OECD. According to the OECD, Portugal is one of the OECD countries with the fewest discharges per 1,000 inhabitants (120), far behind countries like Austria, France and Bulgaria, with figures of 267, 264 and 239, respectively. In other words, although there is a large influx to health services, this doesn't seem to be materialized in a significant number of hospitalizations. This may be the result of low/unsatisfactory coverage by family doctors or unsuccessful regulation of access (low user fees/many exemptions). According to Elliot et al. (2000), although areas of higher population density are associated with greater use of hospitals, this does not translate into a reduction in mortality in these regions, which suggests that perhaps health services would have more impact in another geographic and/or demographic context. This means that the architecture of the hospital network could have a greater impact on population longevity if it took into account factors other than population. After all this background, the following subsections will look at the dynamics of supply and demand in the particular case of nursing.

1.5.3 - DEMAND AND SUPPLY OF NURSING PROFESSIONALS

There has been little scientific literature on the disparity between supply and demand for nurses. It is therefore not easy to pinpoint the ideal number of nurses that a country should have, but it is possible to list the decisive factors that affect the supply of and demand for nurses.

According to Simoens et al. (2005) the demand for nurses tends to increase with population growth, economic expansion, scientific advances, an ageing population and

---

32 Discharge is understood as the situation that occurs when the doctor considers that the treatment provided to the patient during hospitalization has been successful and, as such, authorizes the patient to return home (Webster's New World Medical Dicionary, 2011).

rising patient expectations. With regard to the specific factors influencing the supply of nursing professionals, socio-economic factors such as the ageing of nurses, their early retirement, the country's economic willingness to provide better working conditions, the number of vacancies in schools and the (more or less) attractive salaries offered to nurses stand out. Several studies have looked at these general aspects, as described below.

A study by Simoens et al. (2005) estimated the age distribution of nurses between 2011 and 2021 in countries such as Austria, Belgium, France, Germany, Italy and the Netherlands, concluding that the proportion of nurses under the age of 40 would decrease and that nurses over the age of 45 would increase. This situation will have a negative impact on the supply of nurses in the short/medium term, as mentioned by Aiken and Cheung (2008) and Budge et al. (2003), since it could lead to a shortage of these professionals. On the other hand, studies by Manton, Corder and Stallard (1997) and Reinhart (2003) state that the ageing of the population will have little impact on the demand for health care, since we have to take into account the increase in average life expectancy and the associated increase in quality of life. In other words, this opinion seems to contradict what is commonly believed, based on common sense, that the longer a person's average life expectancy, the more health care they will need, leading to a greater demand for care.

Several authors (Bloor & Maynard, 2003; Birch, O'Brien-Palas, Alksnis, Murphy & Thompson, 2003) have denounced the inability of most countries to adapt their healthcare provision to the changes taking place at social, demographic and even cultural level. These authors also found that when countries did have this concern, it was only focused on doctors and technological/scientific developments. For Tierney (2003), the shortage of nurses is a global problem, but one that can be solved by thinking locally. The author clearly points out the need to hire nurses who are native to the area covered by the hospitals so that they can settle more easily and, as such, don't tend to "flee" the more rural areas. These are the areas that generally have a shortage of these professionals. According to Simoens et al. (2005), another factor leading to a reduction in the supply of health care is the reduction in the number of hours nurses actually work. This decrease in actual working hours may be due to government impositions (a reduction in the number of overtime hours and therefore less availability of services), an increase in part-time work (for example, the accumulation of other functions such as teaching in health schools, training and other activities) and an increase in the number of leisure hours spent by nurses (given their satisfaction with their basic salary).

An article by Berlinier and Ginzberg (2002) and another by Janiszewski (2003) point out that, in the USA, the shortage of nurses, which has already been mentioned, is a phenomenon that follows a cyclical pattern, which had already occurred in the 50s, 70s and 80s of the 20th century. During these periods, the shortage was solved with better pay and benefits, as well as incentives to immigrate. However, Barigozzi and Turati (2010) argue that, in the most serious cases of shortage of nurses, increasing salaries may not be enough, so the solution to the problem must lie in incentives for immigration. For Berlinier and Ginzberg (2002), the shortage predicted for 2010 will not be so easily resolved if decision-makers do not take into account three crucial aspects: (1) removing obstacles to access to the profession, (2) promoting the retention of professionals in the area (by creating incentives, training, etc.) and (3) implementing policies to discourage early retirement.

For all the above reasons, with regard to the actual supply of nurses, it can be concluded that this can be affected by the wealth generated in the country, by variations in the remuneration and productivity of nurses, by the conditions of the health services, by recruitment policies and by a policy of increasing the responsibility of nurses (Simoens et al., 2005). With regard to the graphical representation of the supply and demand of nurses, it can be seen in Figure 6 that for two countries (A and B), a shortage or surplus of nurses can occur if salaries are set at different levels (Pc) from those determined by the intersection of the supply (S) and demand (D) of nurses[33], in a given market.

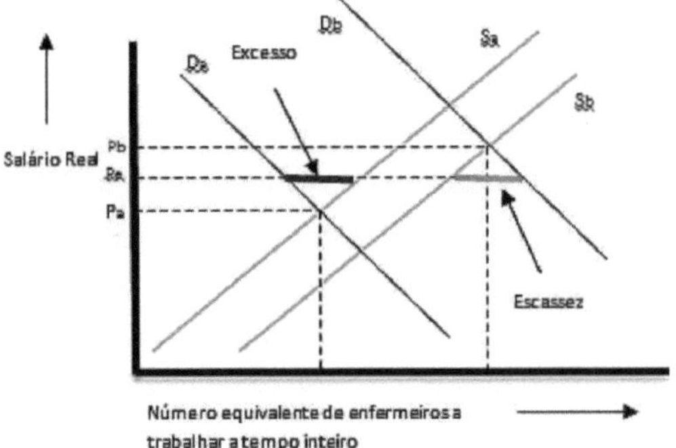

Figura 6. Dynamics of supply and demand for nurses in two countries (A and B) and market consequences when a common price (Pc) is established

Source: Adapted from Simoens et al. (2005, p. 15)

33 This diagram assumes that there is no migration of nurses between two countries in response to wage differences between them.

Figure 6 shows that, theoretically, in country A, nurses' salaries are determined by the intersection of the supply and demand curves, correspondingly Sa and Da. The same is true of country B, except that the nurses' salaries resulting from the intersection of the supply and demand curves are higher than in country A, due to the rightward shift of the Db curve (demand for nurses in country B) being considerably greater than the Sb curve (supply of nurses in country B). This model argues that if the price (Pc) is not determined by the intersections of the supply and demand curves and there is no migration of nurses between these two countries, what will happen is that in country A, there will be a surplus of nurses (represented in dark blue), while in country B, there will be a shortage of nurses (represented in light blue). This is easy to observe in country A since, for a given price Pc, it will first intersect the demand curve for nurses (Da) and only then the supply curve for nurses (Sa). In other words, the quantity of nurses demanded, for this price (Pc), is less than the quantity supplied, hence the surplus of nurses. The opposite situation is seen in country B, since for Pc, it first intersects the supply curve for nurses (Sb) and only then the demand curve (Db), meaning that the quantity of nurses needed is less than the quantity demanded, hence the shortage.

As we have seen above, several authors refer to high levels of demand for nursing care (Bloor & Maynard, 2003; Birch, O'Brien-Palas, Alksnis, Murphy & Thompson, 2003), so a lower supply of nurses can lead to a shortage of nurses if there is no increase in their salaries in line with the supply and demand curves, according to the theoretical model presented here. It should be noted that, although most of the authors cited agree that increasing pay is effective in increasing the supply of nurses, Heyes (2005) argues that it can have negative consequences. The author points out that increasing pay can lead to people being attracted to the nursing profession for the money and not for their vocation[34] . Following on from this study, Taylor (2007) showed that increasing nurses' salaries to combat shortages would be a logical process in a market operating in perfect competition. However, in an NHS characterized by monopsony[35] their salaries would tend to fall[36] which is currently the case, given that the majority employer - the state - continues to tend not to recruit staff and to lower hourly wages. Barigozzi and Turati (2010) argue that the situation is not so straightforward, as they point out that an increase in remuneration could lead, on the one hand, to a decrease in the productivity of nurses without a vocation, but

34 As was discussed in detail in point 1.2.1, when we looked at the deontology of nurses.

35 In economics, monopsony is a form of market with only one buyer and numerous sellers. It is a type of imperfect competition, unlike monopoly, where there is only one seller and several buyers.

36 For example, in Portugal there are only public and private health institutions (which essentially depend on the public sector), and since they dominate the market, they can control wages, in this case by lowering them.

on the other, it could contribute to an increase in the productivity of nurses with a vocation. This thought confirms that of Antonazzo, Scott, Skatun and Elliot (2003) who argue that what directly influences the supply of nurses is their job satisfaction, both in terms of the profession itself and the work environment and hierarchy (Berlinier & Ginzberg, 2002; Barigozzi & Turati, 2010).

In a Government of Canada report called The *International Nursing Labor Market* (Baumann et al., 2004), it is stated that the supply of nurses depends on market forces that have cyclical characteristics. These forces are essentially demographic changes, technological evolution and globalization. Changes in demographics alter the demand for nurses, in line with the needs of the population, but can simultaneously alter supply due, for example, to the ageing of the workforce employed in the nursing sector. Technology affects where and how nurses care for patients and globalization affects their mobility.

In some hospitals, in order to combat the difficulty of deciding how many nurses are actually needed in the services, a nurse per bed ratio is established as a mechanism for regulating the supply of vacancies for nurses (Bloor & Maynard, 2003). The following subsection discusses this issue in more detail and how the indicator influences the demand for nurses.

1.5.4 - NURSE TO PATIENT RATIO AND DISTRIBUTION OF NURSES

Generally speaking, there is no standard ratio for the number of nurses per patient. However, some studies have tried to calculate this ratio for intensive care. In the USA, a study by Pronovost et al. (2001) states that there is a minimum ratio of one nurse to one patient in intensive care units, and this ratio has been established as the ideal provision of care in those circumstances. However, in a study by Zurn, Dal Poz, Stilwell and Adams (2002), the high degree of subjectivity in the task of assigning an ideal number of nurses per patient is admitted, since demand in intensive care units generally fluctuates greatly[37] . It should be noted that, according to Bloor and Maynard (2003), this ratio is different in Australia (1.4), France (0.5), Germany (0.6) and the United Kingdom (1.0).

What seems clear is that the lack of nurses in services leads to an increase in the number of users per nurse, which harms the health of patients (for example, through a lack of attention and control on the part of professionals) and professionals (in the form of physical and/or mental exhaustion, which can lead to *burnout*, for example) (Aiken et al., 2002). Nevertheless, in recent years there has been a tendency on the part of hospital

37 The demand for care in this type of service depends on unpredictable phenomena such as accidents. It is therefore difficult to predict the percentage of occupancy and, therefore, the number of nurses to be assigned.

administrations to reduce the number of beds and the number of days spent in hospital, increasing the number of outpatient surgeries (CNADCA, 2009). This situation has a negative impact on the demand for nursing care since, in principle, fewer nurses will be needed (Pronovost et al., 2001). On the other hand, the increase in average life expectancy, medical-technological advances and investment in long-term/palliative care have made it possible to prolong the lives of patients who, in the past, would not have been able to live as many years (OECD, 2011b), which has a positive influence on the demand for nurses.

The work of Finlayson, Dixon, Meadow and Blair (2002) reveals a different perspective. According to these authors, a shortage of nursing care does not imply a shortage of nurses. In other words, the authors question whether this is a problem of numbers or of the allocation/use of resources. According to them, we will only really know where and to what extent there is a shortage of nurses if they all stop working at the same time, and then we can survey the extent of the needs in each service.

While it is possible to find literature on the supply and demand of doctors in Portugal, it has been more difficult to find research on the distribution of nurses. In the case of doctors, Correia and Veiga's (2009) study describes major disparities in the distribution of doctors, mainly due to inequities in salary distribution, despite the number of doctors being above the OECD average (OECD, 2011b). In the case of nursing, however, and despite various existing statistics, particularly from the National Institute of Statistics and the Order of Nurses, there is no known study looking at the distribution of nurses in Portugal and the respective reasons for their distribution. Therefore, the research work proposed here aims to add value to the analysis of this problem by adding to the traditional descriptive analysis of the data the respective framework with the reality of the other OECD countries, adding econometric analysis methods that better explain the geographical distribution of nurses, their respective motivations and the factors that influence this distribution. To this end, the aim is to use variables that are considered empirically important for analyzing the distribution of nurses and to see if there is a relationship between them and the distribution that is found.

Internationally, there have been a few studies on this subject, although they are scarce. In particular, the study by Lin et al. (1997) shows that there is a higher concentration of nurses in urban areas, and that this concentration is positively related to that of doctors. Studies by Wong et al. (2009) show that the geographical distribution of primary health care nurses is similar to that of doctors and is not related to the health status of the population covered. As for nurses' motivations for choosing regions (more rural or more urban), according to Skillman et al. (2005) and Henwood et al. (2009), nurses working in rural areas tend to earn lower salaries and work longer hours, due to the smaller supply of nurses. They tend to have lower qualifications than nurses working in urban areas and are more inclined to move to other areas. Both studies call for policies specifically targeted at rural areas to make them more attractive to this type of professional, thus making a strong contribution to combating desertification.

Since the aim of this work is to observe and analyze the distribution of nurses at the municipal level, describing and explaining their possible motivations, the following chapter is divided into two sub-sections: The first aims to provide a statistical framework of the nursing profession in Portugal and in a selection of OECD countries in their various contexts, also seeking to compare this reality with the economic and health data of these same countries. The second sub-section aims to carry out an econometric analysis of the distribution of nurses in Portugal at county level, using the Gini coefficient to check the equity of distribution of these health professionals and the OLS methodology in order to understand which variables influence the distribution of nurses for the years 2002, 2010 and the respective variation between the two periods.

CHAPTER II

DESCRIPTIVE AND INFERENTIAL STATISTICAL ANALYSIS OF THE DISTRIBUTION OF NURSES

2.1. DESCRIPTIVE STATISTICAL ANALYSIS

In this work, in order to provide a better understanding, it was decided to divide this chapter into two parts: descriptive statistical analysis and inferential analysis. We decided to do this because they are two important aspects, but they should be analyzed separately. This sub-chapter will analyze all the statistical data relating to nurses in Portugal, putting it into context with the world (OECD countries), without ever neglecting the reality and the economic and health development of each of them. In this way, the aim is to situate the figures relating to these professionals in relation to the other countries, verifying their position in relation to them.

Once the statistical framework of Portugal has been established, an analysis will be made of the interior of the country, looking at the differences or asymmetries between the various districts of Portugal. There will also be a more detailed analysis of the numbers of nurses in Portugal, considering their evolution over time, exploring the possible causes of increases or decreases.

2.1.1. national and international framework for statistical information on the number of nurses in portugal

The aim of this section is to contextualize the situation of nurses in Portugal, comparing them, from an international perspective, with other European countries and, from a national perspective, moving on to a more detailed analysis of the data available for the Portuguese economy. However, before presenting and analyzing the statistical data on nurses in Portugal, it is important to provide a statistical framework for the evolution of both health expenditure and some health indicators, in order to better understand the context of the Health System in Portugal. The table below (Table 3) shows some of Portugal's economic and health indicators and their respective evolution from 1970 to 2009. These indicators are: total health expenditure as a percentage of GDP and *per capita* expenditure. This data is important to know what percentage of the country's wealth is invested in health and how much money is involved, as each country has its own GDP. It was decided to also include the number of doctors and consultations per capita, due to the complementarity and proportionality that the work of nurses has with doctors. The items total hospital beds, hospital discharges and average days in hospital serve to give an idea of how the hospital works, both in terms of workflows and routines, and are indicators that, according to the OECD (OECD, 2011b), characterize the health policies of each country, as we have already seen earlier in this dissertation. Finally, according to the same organization, the indicators of average life expectancy and mortality rate are classic indicators of the state of health of countries and even of the development of countries.

Table 3

Evolution of health indicators in Portugal from 1970-2009

Health indicators■	Year									Average growth rate (1970-2009*) (%)
	1970	1975	1980	1985	1990	1995	2000	2005	2009*	
Total health expenditure (% GDP)	2,4	5	5,1	5,6	5,7	7,5	9,3	10,4	10,1	3,85
Total health expenditure per capita (US$)	47	158	277	395	628	1.014	1.654	2.212	2.508	11,03
Doctors (1,000hab)	0,9	1,2	2	2,5	2,8	2,9	3,2	3,4	3,8	3,67
Total Hospital beds (per 1,000 inhabitants)				4	4	3,9	3,8	3,5	3,3	
No. of consultations per capita	2	3,1	3,7	2,8	3	3,2	3,5	3,9	4,1	1,86
Hospital discharges (per 100,000 inhabitants)						8.740	8.622	9.066	11.250	
Average number of days in hospital	15,3	12,5	11,4	11,1	8,4	7,9	7,7	7,1	6,7	-2,10
Average life expectancy	66,7	68,4	71,4	73	74,1	75,4	76,7	78,1	79,5	0,45
Infant mortality rate (per 1,000 births)	55,5	38,9	24,3	17,8	10,9	7,4	5,5	3,5	3,6	-6,77

Notes:* Data for 2009 or the closest year with available data. The only data for 2008 is total expenditure and *per capita* expenditure on health.

Source: Own elaboration based on data collected in *OECD Health Data 2011*.

As can be seen in the table, Portugal shows an upward trend in the percentage of GDP spent on health expenditure. The figures rise from 2.4% in 1970 to a maximum of 10.4% in 2005, falling slightly to 10.1% in 2008, the last year for which information is available. Even so, during this period there was an average growth rate of 3.85%. At the same time, total health expenditure *per capita* went from 47 US dollars in 1970, growing exponentially to 2,508 US dollars in 2010. This figure corresponds to an average growth rate of 11.03% per year in the amount spent on health per Portuguese citizen, which is quite significant. This increase in individual investment in health was accompanied by an increase in the number of doctors per thousand inhabitants. This number increased from 0.9 doctors per thousand inhabitants in 1970 to 3.9 in 2010, which represents an average increase of 3.67% per year over a 40-year period. There has also been a general increase in consultations per doctor (1.86% per year on average) and in the number of hospital discharges, which indicates an increase in the use of healthcare. The same is not true of the number of hospital beds, which is showing a downward trend, and the average number of days spent in hospital, which has fallen by an average of 2.10% a year. The latter indicator has been on a downward trend, mainly due to scientific developments in the hospital sector and policies to encourage outpatient surgery, which aim to improve the patient's quality of life and reduce hospital costs (CNADCA, 2009). All these factors have made an important contribution to the huge increase in average life expectancy in Portugal - from 66.7 years in 1970 to 79.5 in 2009 - and to a notable reduction in infant mortality - from 55.5 per 1,000 births in 1970 to 3.6 in 2009, representing a decrease of 6.77% per year on average.

Having analyzed Portugal's development from 1970 to 2009 in terms of some of the most important internationally comparable health indicators, it is also important to understand how it compares statistically with some of the OECD countries[38] in 2009 (the last year for which statistically comparable information is available). It should be remembered that the OECD is made up of the most developed countries in the world. The following table (Table 4) shows the same indicators presented for Portugal in the previous table, but only for 2009.

Table 4

Health indicators in Portugal and some OECD countries in 2009

Indicators	Year								
	Poland	Spain	Estonia	Denmark	Hungary	USA	Slovakia	Ireland	Portugal
GDP *per capita* (US$)	18.924	32.146	19.789	38.229	20.154	45.087	22.581	39.750	24.935
Total health expenditure (% GDP)	7,4	9,5	7	11,5	7,4	17,4	9,1	9,5	10,1 (1)
Total health expenditure per capita (US$)	1.394	3.067	1.393	4.348	1.511	7.960	2.084	3.781	2.508 (1)
Out of Pocket Payments	310	616	282	573	359	976	533	464	681 (1)

38 A comparison with these countries was chosen because it was felt that a better comparison with Portugal could be made by selecting countries with a higher Gross Domestic Product (GDP) than Portugal, such as Ireland, Denmark, Spain and the USA, and countries with a lower GDP than Portugal, such as Poland, Hungary, Estonia and Slovakia.

Doctors (per 1,000 inhabitants)	2,2	3,5	3,3	3,4 (1)	3	2,4	3 (3)	3,1	3,8
Total Hospital beds (per 1,000 inhabitants)	6,7	3,2	5,4	3,5	7,1	3,1	6,5	4,9 (1)	3,3
No. of consultations per capita	6,8	7,5	6,3	4,6	12	3,9 (1)	12,1 (1)	3,3 (2)	4,1
Hospital discharges (per 100,000 inhabitants)	20.107	10.411	16.984	17.032	18.502	13.086 (1)	21.100	13.236	11.250
Average number of days in hospital	4	3	-	2,7	4,5	2,1 (1)	5,4	2,1	2,7
Average life expectancy	76	82	75	79	74	78,2	75	80	79,5
Infant mortality rate (per 1,000 births)	5,6	3,3	3,6	3,1	5,1	6,5 (1)	5,7	3,2	3,6

Note: (1) 2008 figures, (2) 2007 figures and (3) 2006 figures.

Source: Own elaboration based on data collected in OECD *Health Data* 2011.

Table 4 shows the values of some health expenditure and health care indicators for some OECD countries. The country with the highest percentage of GDP allocated to health is the USA. It spends 17.4% of the wealth it generates on health. It is followed by Denmark with 11.5% and Portugal with 10.1%. In terms of health expenditure *per capita,* Portugal only spends 2,508 US dollars per individual, well below the US, which spends 7,960 US dollars per individual, and Denmark and Ireland, which spend 4,348 and 3,781 US dollars per individual, respectively. More specifically, with regard to expenditure borne directly by individuals, *out of pocket expenditure,* the countries with the highest figures are the USA (976 dollars), followed by Portugal (681 dollars) and Spain (616 dollars). The lowest values for *out-of-pocket* payments are in Estonia (282 dollars), Poland (310 dollars) and Hungary (359 dollars). According to the literature consulted, in particular the work by Ku and his co-authors (2003), an increase in the percentage of *out-of-pocket* payments in a given country may indicate that the country's health system is weak in terms of the quality and coverage of public health care provided to the population. When this happens, the population has to spend more of its own money when seeking health care. An opposing view is presented by Plumper and Neumeyer (2012). These authors argue that an increase in the percentage of *out-of-pocket* payments will contribute to a decrease in the mortality rate. For example, by limiting unnecessary visits to emergency departments, they can focus more specifically on truly urgent situations, which in turn reduces hospital mortality rates.

With regard to the number of doctors per thousand inhabitants shown in table 4, the country with the highest figures in 2009 is Portugal, with 3.8 doctors per thousand inhabitants. Poland and the USA had the lowest figures, 2.2 and 2.4 doctors per thousand inhabitants respectively. Also noteworthy is the fact that the number of hospital beds is highest in Poland and Hungary (6.7 and 7.1 respectively) while Portugal has the lowest (3.3). This factor also seems to lead to the number of discharges per thousand inhabitants in Portugal being one of the lowest - 11,250 per 1,000 inhabitants. An interesting fact is the number of consultations *per capita. These are* highest in Slovakia and Hungary, at 12.1 and 12 respectively, while in countries such as Ireland (3.3), the USA (3.9) and Portugal (4.1) they are considerably lower. These figures are even more interesting if they are compared with those relating to the number of doctors per thousand inhabitants, health expenditure and *out of pocket payments* made in these countries. In addition to the above figures, Portugal is one of the countries with the highest life expectancy for its entire population - 79.5 years (OECD, 2001a).

After providing a statistical framework for Portugal, in terms of health indicators, in relation to a selected set of OECD countries, with the highest and lowest wealth generated in 2009, and having understood the evolution of these indicators over time for the Portuguese economy, we will begin the analysis of the object of study of this research work - nurses. It is believed that with the framework provided, it will be possible to gain a better understanding of the statistical data on the number of nurses that will be presented below.

Figure 7 compares the number of nurses per thousand inhabitants in Portugal with the total number of OECD countries. As mentioned above, this comparison allows the object of this research to be contextualized from an international perspective.

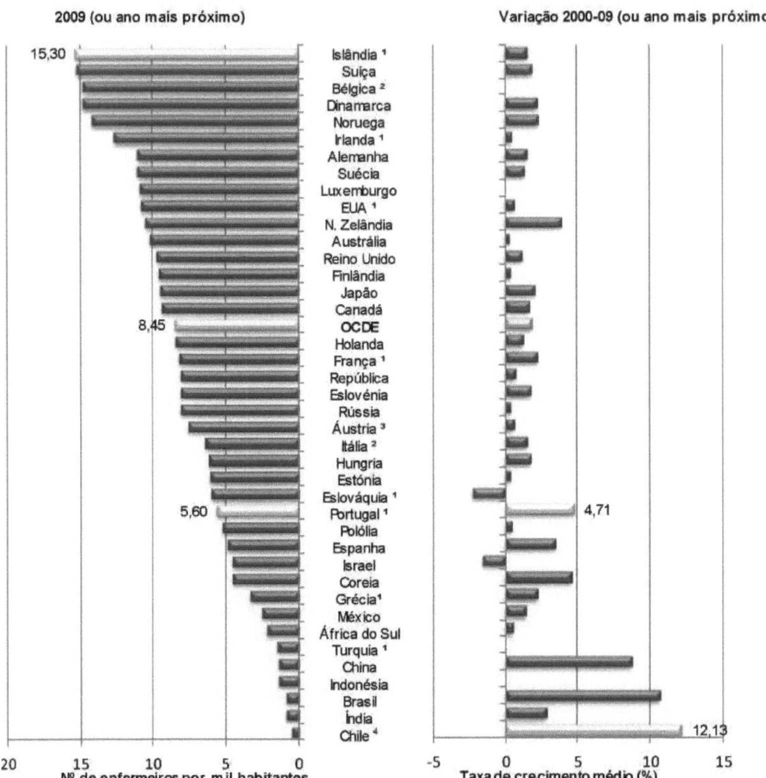

Notes: 1) The data includes not only nurses who provide direct care to patients, but also those who work in the management of health units, education, research, etc.; 2) The data refers to all nurses with a license to practice; 3) Austria only reports nurses who work in hospitals; 4) Chile only includes nurses who work in the public sector.

Figura 7. Number of nurses per thousand inhabitants in OECD countries in 2009 and their average annual growth over the period 2000-2009

Source: Adapted from OECD Health Data 2011; WHO-Europe for the Russian Federation and national sources for other nonOECD countries.

The figure above shows that the country with the highest number of nurses per 1,000 inhabitants is Iceland, with 15.30 nurses per thousand inhabitants. The country with the lowest figure is Chile with only 0.9 nurses per thousand inhabitants. Portugal has 5.60 nurses per 1,000 inhabitants, below the OECD average of 8.45 nurses per 1,000 inhabitants. However, Portugal's average growth rate over the 9-year period under analysis, which corresponds to the first decade of this century, is significant - the number of nurses in Portugal (per thousand inhabitants) grew by an average of 4.7% per year. This figure indicates that, although the number of nurses in Portugal is still somewhat below the OECD average, it is showing an upward trend in terms of the number of nurses, especially when compared to countries with a higher density of nurses than its own. The country with the highest average annual growth rate over the period is Chile (12.1%). Chile, despite being the country with the fewest nurses per thousand inhabitants, seems to be making efforts to counteract this trend. The only two countries with negative average annual growth rates over the period are Slovakia (-2.3%) and Israel (-1.6%).

It is also interesting to see how many nurses there are in Portugal and in some OECD countries, in relation to the existing workforce in each of them. The figure below (Figure 8) shows the number of nursing graduates per thousand active nurses in Portugal and the other OECD countries in 2009.

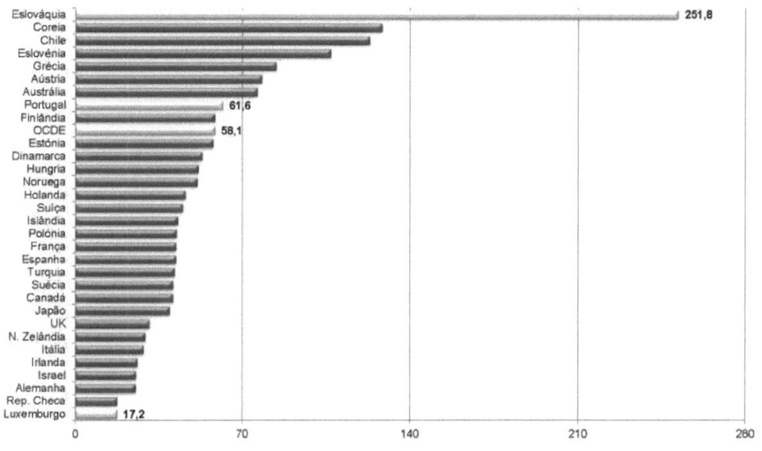

Figura 8. Number of nursing graduates per 1,000 active nurses in 2009[39] , in OECD countries

Source: Adapted from OECD Health at a Glance 2011. http://dx.doi.org/1001787/88893524336

As can be seen in the figure above, in 2009 Portugal had 61.6 new nurses for every thousand existing nurses, which is above countries like Germany, the United Kingdom and

39 Or the closest year with statistical information available.

even above the average for OECD countries - 58.1 new nurses trained for every thousand existing nurses. Slovakia is the country with the most nurses trained (251.18) per thousand existing nurses in 2009, and Luxembourg has the lowest number (17.2).

It is also interesting to look at the number of nursing graduates per 100,000 inhabitants, in order to clarify the weight of new nurses in the existing population in each country. This indicator is shown in Figure 9, which compares the different countries that make up the OECD.

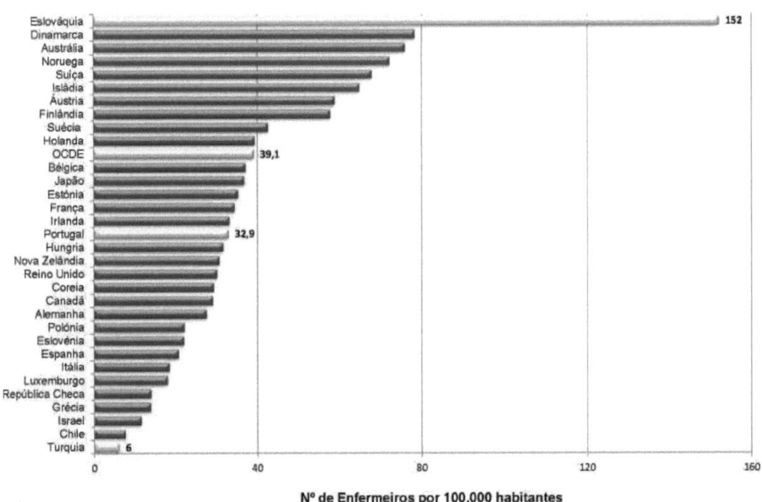

Figura 9. Number of nursing graduates per 100,000 inhabitants in OECD countries in 2009

Source: Adapted from OECD Health at a Glance 2011. http://dx.doi.org/10.1787/888932524317

In Portugal, the number of trained nurses per 100,000 inhabitants in 2009 is below the OECD average (39.1), with 32.9 trained nurses per 100,000 inhabitants. This figure is still above countries such as Germany, Spain, Greece and Canada and far below countries such as Slovakia (152), Denmark (78.3) and Australia (75.9).

After looking at the data for 2009, it is important to check the evolution of the number of graduate nurses per 100,000 inhabitants between 1998 and 2008 in some OECD countries[40] in order to get an idea of their evolutionary curve. The following tables (Table 5 and Table 6) show the statistical data relating to this evolution, as well as the respective

40 These countries were selected because three of them have a higher GDP *per capita* than Portugal - Denmark, Ireland and Finland - and the other three have a lower GDP *per capita* than Portugal - Poland, Slovakia and Estonia.

average annual growth rates over the period and the annual growth rate of the same indicator.

Evolution of the number of graduate nurses per 100,000 inhabitants, from 1998 to 2008, in a selected group of OECD countries .[41]

Countries	Year											
	1998	1999	2000	2001	2002	2003	2004	2005	2006	2007	2008	Average growth rate (%)
Denmark	100,1	104,7	101,0	99,7	103,5	77,3	81,9	78,1	80,3	78,8	78,3	-2,43
Estonia	20,9	5,1	20,1	24,0	29,8	32,2	28,9	35,9	35,0	44,0	28,1	3,00
Finland	86,0	79,1	69,0	61,6	59,3	51,4	47,8	44,8	46,6	49,8	56,1	-4,18
Ireland	36,8	40,2	38,6	26,6	31,4	30,4	44,4	34,5	35,6	32,5	35,5	-0,36
Portugal	14,1	16,1	16,8	18,7	4,0	17,6	21,0	28,0	32,5	33,4	32,9	8,84
Poland	0,8	1,1	1,1	1,8	2,4	2,5	4,3	7,1	18,2	20,8	24,1	40,57
Slovakia	49,8	55,7	53,8	49,5	51,8	41,2	61,0	32,1	69,2	85,6	114,3	8,66

Source: Own elaboration based on data from *OECD Health Data 2011*

Table 6

Evolution of the annual growth rate in the number of graduate nurses per 100,000 inhabitants, from 1998 to 2008, in a selected group of OECD countries (%).

Countries	Year									
	1999	2000	2001	2002	2003	2004	2005	2006	2007	2008
Denmark	4,60	-3,53	-1,29	3,81	-25,31	5,95	-4,64	2,82	-1,87	-0,63
Estonia	-75,60	294,12	19,40	24,17	8,05	-10,25	24,22	-2,51	25,71	-36,14
Finland	-8,02	-12,77	-10,72	-3,73	-13,32	-7,00	-6,28	4,02	6,87	12,65
Ireland	9,24	-3,98	-31,09	18,05	-3,18	46,05	-22,30	3,19	-8,71	9,23
Portugal	14,18	4,35	11,31	-78,61	340,00	19,32	33,33	16,07	2,77	-1,50
Poland	37,50	0,00	63,64	33,33	4,17	72,00	65,12	156,34	14,29	15,87
Slovakia	11,85	-3,41	-7,99	4,65	-20,46	48,06	-47,38	115,58	23,70	33,53

Source: Own elaboration based on data from *OECD Health Data 2011*

As can be seen in Table 5, Portugal went from 14.1 graduate nurses per 100,000 inhabitants in 1998 to 32.9 in 2008, which represents an average annual increase of 8.84% over the period. In relative terms, Poland stands out, with an average increase of 40.57% per year. Other countries, such as Denmark and Finland, recorded an average annual decrease in the number of graduate nurses per 100,000 inhabitants. In terms of the annual growth rate over the same period, Portugal has seen solid growth. There have

41

been increases in most years, especially the sharp increase of 340% in 2003 (compared to 2002) and the decreases in 2002 and 2008. It should be noted that while Portugal shows a constant trend of annual growth, countries such as Ireland, Denmark and Finland seem to alternate between annual increases and decreases, which may indicate the existence of some self-regulation mechanisms in the supply of these professionals.

As mentioned earlier in this dissertation, the work of nurses is directly influenced by the work of doctors (Lin et al., 1997; Budge et al., 2003), particularly in terms of prescribing. It is therefore pertinent to look at how many nurses are available for each active doctor. The latest available figures for the indicator relating to the ratio of nurses to doctors in 2009 can be seen, both for Portugal and for the other OECD countries, in the next figure (Figure 10).

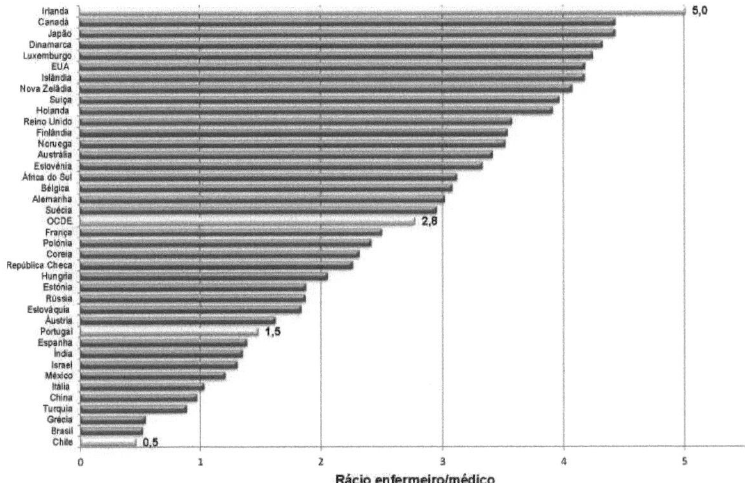

Figura 10. : Ratio of nurses to doctors in a selection[42] of OECD countries in 2009 (or nearest available year).

Source: Adapted from OECD Health data 2011. http://dx.doi.org/10.1787/888325524298

Figure 10 shows that, in 2009, Portugal had a ratio of 1.5 nurses per doctor - for every two doctors working, there were 3 nurses available. As you can see, this figure is far from the OECD average of 2.8 nurses per doctor. The figure is even further away from that of the country with the highest ratio - Ireland - with 5 nurses per doctor. There are, however, countries with the opposite trend to most of the countries under analysis, for example Chile

42 It was decided to select only those countries for which data was available for 2009 on the number of doctors and nurses. The average shown corresponds to the average of the countries in the figure.

has a ratio of 0.5 nurses per doctor, which means that for every two doctors working there is only one nurse.

After analyzing the information on some indicators related to the subject under study, from an international perspective, information on the number of nurses in the Portuguese economy will be analyzed. To begin this analysis, we present the distribution of the number of nurses in 2010, by Portuguese district, in absolute and percentage terms (Figure 11).

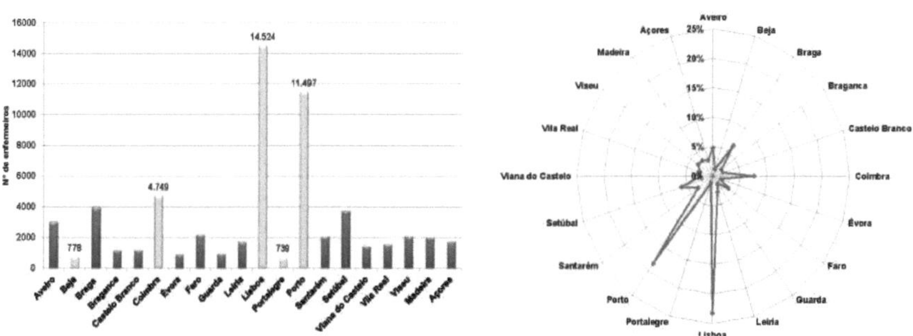

Figura 11. Number of nurses in Portugal in absolute and percentage terms, by district, in 2010

Source: Ordem dos Enfermeiros statistical data 2000-2010.

The figure above shows that the districts where there are clearly the most nurses in absolute terms are Lisbon (with 14,524 nurses), Porto (11,497) and Coimbra (4,749), which are clearly the most predominant districts in terms of percentage of nurses - these three districts account for 49% of the total number of nurses in Portugal. At the other extreme are Portalegre (739) and Beja (778). This study will examine whether these results are influenced by the distribution of the Portuguese population by district or whether they are not. In order to cancel out the population effect, the number of nurses per thousand inhabitants for the same period and for the same geographical location is shown below in visual form (Figure 12).

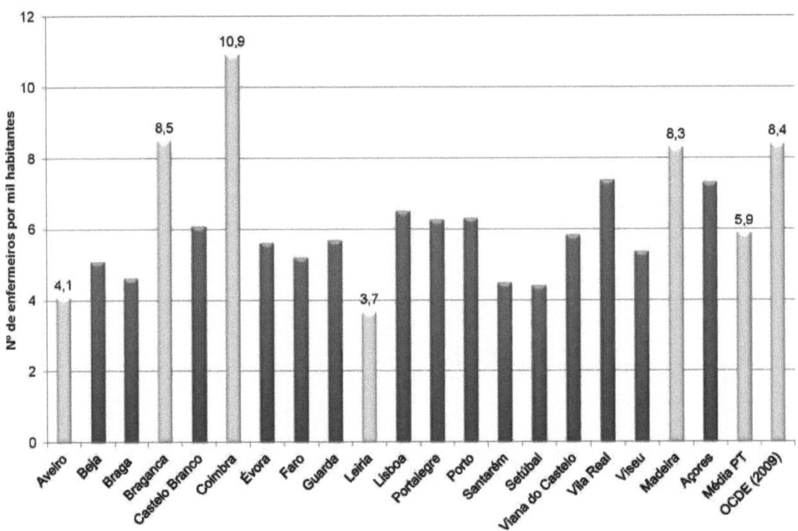

Figure 12 : Number of nurses per thousand inhabitants in Portugal, by district, in 2010

Source: Ordem dos Enfermeiros statistical data 2000-2010.

Taking out the population effect, the data shows a very different picture. As for the number of nurses per thousand inhabitants, in the 18 Portuguese districts, the ones with the highest values are Coimbra (with 10.9 nurses per thousand inhabitants), Bragança (8.5) and the Autonomous Region of Madeira (8.3). Although these districts have the highest figures for the indicator, only Coimbra and Bragança are above the OECD average for 2009 - 8.5 nurses per thousand inhabitants. At the other end of the spectrum, at less than half the OECD average, are the districts of Leiria and Aveiro, with only 3.7 and 4.1 nurses per thousand inhabitants, respectively. It should be noted that the average number of nurses per thousand inhabitants in Portugal is 5.9, well below the 8.5 mentioned above as the average for OECD countries.

In order to give an idea of how the number of nurses in the different Portuguese districts has evolved, Figure 13 shows the variation in the total number of nurses per district between 2001 and 2010. The right-hand side of the graph also shows the absolute percentage change in the number of nurses in each district over the 10-year period under analysis.

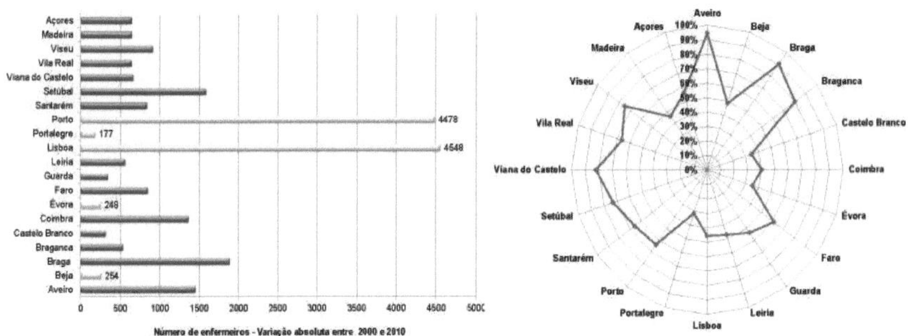

Figura 13 Absolute and percentage change in the total number of nurses, by district, between 2001 and 2010

Source: Ordem dos Enfermeiros statistical data 2000-2010.

Between 2001 and 2010 there was an increase in the number of nurses in all the districts of mainland Portugal and the islands. This increase was most pronounced in the districts of Lisbon and Porto, with increases of over 4,000 nurses. However, it is interesting to note that in percentage terms the districts with the biggest increase in nurses between 2001 and 2010 were Aveiro, Braga and Viana do Castelo. On the other hand, in percentage terms, the districts with the smallest increases were Portalegre, Castelo Branco and Évora. The districts of Portalegre and Évora saw increases of only 177 and 248 nurses, respectively, between 2001 and 2010. With this data, we can see that although there was a greater increase in the absolute number of nurses in Lisbon and Porto, the districts where there was a greater effort to integrate these professionals were Aveiro, Braga and Viana do Castelo, and in Aveiro these professionals almost doubled between 2001 and 2010. On the negative side, Portalegre and Beja stand out as the districts with the smallest increase in the absolute number of nurses and also the smallest percentage change over the period.

As presented in the previous chapter, it is important to note that a nurse can have different levels of specialization, so there are generalist and specialist nurses. The following table shows the distribution of the number of nurses by specialty, as in the previous chapter, but in greater detail as it also includes the annual and average growth rates for each period, as well as the respective evolution between 2000 and 2010.

Table 7

Distribution and evolution of the number of generalist and specialist nurses in Portugal from 2000 to 2010

Specialty-	Year										
	2000	2001	2002	2003	2004	2005	2006	2007	2008	2009	2010
General Nurse	30.883	32.855	35.112	37.182	39.172	41.440	44.069	46.443	48.401	50.040	51.903
Annual growth rate (%)		6,39	6,87	5,90	5,35	5,79	6,34	5,39	4,22	3,39	3,72
Specialist Nurse	6.740	6.794	6.790	6.796	6.734	6.856	7.032	7.785	8.465	9.715	10.673
Annual growth rate (%)		0,80	-0,06	0,09	-0,91	1,81	2,57	10,71	8,73	14,77	9,86
Total	37.623	39.655	41.909	43.984	45.911	48.302	51.107	54.233	56.870	59.758	62.566
Annual **growth rate** (%)		5,40	5,68	4,95	4,38	5,21	5,81	6,12	4,86	5,08	4,70
2000-2010 (%)						5,22					

Source: Adapted from Ordem dos Enfermeiros: statistical data 2000-2010 (OE, 2011f)

As can be seen from the table above, the number of nurses, both generalists and specialists, showed an upward trend between 2000 and 2010, with an annual growth rate for the total number of nurses of between 4.38 and 6.12% and an average growth rate over the period (2000 to 2010) of 5.22%, i.e. relatively stable growth rates. It is interesting to note that the annual growth rates for generalist nurses are much more stable than for specialists. However, the increase in the number of generalist nurses has been decreasing from 2000 to 2010, which could be a sign of containment/regulation policies. In the case of specialist nurses, from 2000 to 2004 the increases in the number of specialists were very small (less than 1%) and alternated with decreases (2202 and 2004). From 2006 onwards, the increase in the number of specialist nurses was considerably higher, which may indicate greater investment by nurses in their academic training.

An analysis by specialty complements the above information. The following table shows the evolution of the absolute distribution of the number of nurses, by specialty, from 2000 to 2010. This data has already been presented in the previous chapter (Table 8), however, it will now be analyzed in greater detail, highlighting the annual and average growth rates for each specialty and each year.

Table 8

Distribution and evolution of the number of nurses, by specialty, in Portugal from 2000 to 2010

Specialty	Year										
	2000	2001	2002	2003	2004	2005	2006	2007	2008	2009	2010

Rehabilitation	1.017	1.023	1.027	1.033	1.029	1.049	1.111	1.233	1.403	1.745	1.962
(%)*		0,59	0,39	0,58	-0,39	1,94	5,91	10,98	13,79	24,38	12,44
Child Health	961	973	978	982	989	987	1.044	1.196	1.314	1.498	1.649
(%)*		1,25	0,51	0,41	0,71	-0,20	5,78	14,56	9,87	14,00	10,08
Maternal Health	1.576	1.576	1.556	1.553	1.516	1.641	1.699	1.898	2.032	2.174	2.329
(%)*		0,00	-1,27	-0,19	-2,38	8,25	3,53	11,71	7,06	6,99	7,13
Public Health	584	576	563	-	-	-	-	-	-	-	-
(%)*		-1,37	-2,26	-	-	-	-	-	-	-	-
Medico-Clinical	1.141	1.157	1.175	1.177	1.176	1.179	1.194	1.275	1.365	1.578	1.767
(%)*		1,40	1,56	0,17	-0,08	0,26	1,27	6,78	7,06	15,60	11,98
Community Health	478	500	513	1.082	1.076	1.069	1.078	1.247	1.349	1.545	1.699
(%)*		4,60	2,60	110,92	-0,55	-0,65	0,84	15,68	8,18	14,53	9,97
Mental Health	983	989	978	969	948	931	906	936	1.002	1.173	1.264
(%)*		0,61	-1,11	-0,92	-2,17	-1,79	-2,69	3,31	7,05	17,07	7,76
Total	6.740	6.794	6.790	6.796	6.734	6.856	7.032	7.785	8.465	9.715	10.673
Annual growth rate of the total (%)		0,80	-0,06	0,09	-0,91	1,81	2,57	10,71	8,73	14,77	9,86
Average growth rate 2000-2010 (%)						4,70					

Notes: * Annual growth rate in % for each age group considered

Source: Own elaboration based on data from Ordem dos Enfermeiros: statistical data 2000-2010 (OE, 2011f).

The table above shows that, between 2000 and 2010, there was a tendency to maintain the number of specialist nurses between 2000 and 2005. The period showed total annual growth rates alternating between positive and negative, never exceeding 1%. Looking specifically at each specialty, we see alternating increases and decreases, with a clear highlight being the increase of more than 110% in the community health specialty in 2003, the same year that the public health specialty ended. As we have seen before, these factors were related, since a large number of public health professionals were integrated into the community health specialty (Graça & Henriques, 2000), which explains this disparate variation.

Still in the same table, from 2006 onwards there was notable growth in all specialties, which continued until 2010. In this second period, total annual growth rates vary between 2.57% and 14.77%. In the specialties in particular, we would highlight the large increases seen, for example in rehabilitation (24%) and mental health (17%), both in 2009. This growth was not unrelated to the increase in the number of schools and the training on offer at existing schools (DGES, 2012), coupled with an increase in nurses' investment in their academic training, possibly due to possible incentives in terms of career progression. In all the years between 2000 and 2010, the annual growth rates correspond to an average growth rate of 4.70% per year.

The following figure (Figure 14) shows the variation in the number of nurses in each specialty from 2000 to 2010, as well as the absolute growth rate of nurses by specialty from 2000 to 2010[43] .

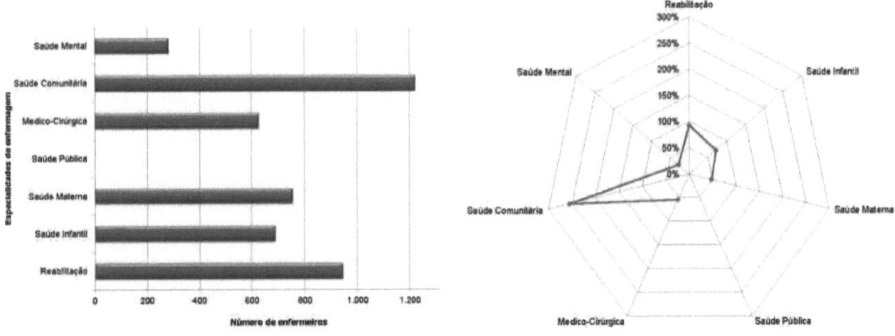

Figura 14 Absolute and percentage increase in the number of nurses, by specialty, between 2000 and 2010

Source: Ordem dos Enfermeiros statistical data 2000-2010.

It's clear to see that the specialties that grew the most were, in descending order: community health, rehabilitation, maternal health, child health, medical-surgical and, finally, mental health. In terms of percentage change, the large increase in the number of professionals with the medical-surgical and rehabilitation specialties stands out, with 255 and 93% increases respectively between 2001 and 2010, which shows a growing interest among nurses in this curricular component. It should be noted that the community health specialty was abolished in 2003, which is why no figures are presented for the period in question.

For a more complete analysis of the number of nurses in Portugal, it is also important to

43 Note that for the public health specialty, no figures are given for the reasons given above.

look at the age distribution of nurses in the Portuguese economy. Above all, the aim is to provide an idea of which age group predominates in the nursing workforce in Portugal and whether or not there could be an adequate regeneration of professionals. In other words, whether there is a risk of a downward trend in the number of nurses due to the fact that the number of retirees may, in the future, be greater than the number of graduates (new nurses). As we saw in Chapter I, several authors such as Berlinier and Ginzberg (2002), Buchan (2002), Budge et al. (2003) and Tierney (2003) state that the shortage of nurses is already a worldwide reality. As such, it is important to check whether there are signs of this happening in Portugal too. We have already seen that the number of nurses per thousand inhabitants and the ratio of nurses to doctors is lower than the OECD average. But in order to see whether the number of nurses could worsen over time, it is of the utmost importance to look at the age distribution of these professionals, as shown in Table 9.

Table 9

Evolution of the number of nurses, by age group, between 2000 and 2010 and respective annual growth rate and average growth over the period

Age group –	Year											Average growth rate (%)
	2000	2001	2002	2003	2004	2005	2006	2007	2008	2009	2010	
21 a 30	6.100	7.829	11.578	12.292	12.917	14.175	15.719	17.456	18.633	20.021	21.043	13,2
(%)*		28,3	47,9	6,2	5,1	9,7	10,9	11,1	6,7	7,4	5,1	
31 a 40	13.325	13.574	13.553	13.861	14.195	14.348	14.560	14.845	15.339	16.201	17.153	2,6
(%)*		1,9	-0,2	2,3	2,4	1,1	1,5	2,0	3,3	5,6	5,9	
41 a 50	8.870	8.986	8.483	9.097	9.741	10.278	10.937	11.520	12.041	12.346	12.800	3,7
(%)*		1,3	-5,6	7,2	7,1	5,5	6,4	5,3	4,5	2,5	3,7	
51 a 60	6.250	6.290	6.017	6.200	6.347	6.587	6.741	7.003	7.218	7.361	7.560	1,9
(%)*		0,6	-4,3	3,0	2,4	3,8	2,3	3,9	3,1	2,0	2,7	
More than 61	3.078	2.973	2.271	2.528	2.706	2.908	3.138	3.396	3.628	3.816	4.010	2,7
(%)*		-3,4	-23,6	11,3	7,0	7,5	7,9	8,2	6,8	5,2	5,1	

Notes: * Annual growth rate in % for each age group considered

Source: Own elaboration based on data from Ordem dos Enfermeiros: statistical data 2000-2010

As can be seen, from 2000 to 2010, there was an increase in the number of nurses in the different age groups illustrated in the figure above, with a special focus on the 21 to 30 age group, i.e. the youngest. In this age group there was an average growth rate of 13.2% from 2000 to 2010, which is quite significant, a far cry from the second age group with the highest average growth rate, which was the 41 to 50 bracket with 3.7%. But even so, all age groups had positive average growth rates, which is to be expected since, as we have already seen, the number of nurses in Portugal has been gradually increasing. Looking at the annual growth rates, they show a general upward trend in all age groups. It is interesting to note that in 2001 and 2002 the 61+ age group saw somewhat sharp declines, but in contrast the 21-30 age group saw strong increases in those same periods, which suggests the existence of some kind of compensatory mechanisms. It is interesting to note that in the remaining periods these two age groups showed very similar growth rates, which shows that the rate at which new nurses enter the workforce is similar to the rate at which they retire. As for the other age groups, the 31 to 40 age group showed a slight upward trend between 2000 and 2010, while the 41 to 50 age group showed a slight downward trend.

2.2. INFERENTIAL ANALYSIS OF THE DISTRIBUTION OF NURSES IN PORTUGAL

2.2.1. ECONOMETRIC METHODOLOGY AND SOURCE OF STATISTICAL DATA

The *Ordinary Least Squares (*OLS) regression methodology (Correia & Veiga, 2010; Lin et al., 1997) will be used to verify which factors explain and influence the number of nurses and their respective geographical distribution in mainland Portugal and the islands. The aim is to understand which socio-demographic variables influence the distribution of nurses in Portugal and to quantify this effect. The number of nurses per thousand inhabitants is the variable to be studied, and the distribution of these health professionals is analyzed at the level of the 308 municipalities in mainland Portugal and the islands. The variables chosen to explain the distribution of nurses, as well as the motivations that led to their choice, will be described in detail below (Table 10). In general terms, the selection of the set of variables that can explain the geographical distribution of nurses in Portugal will follow some of the guidelines presented in the literature review.

The analysis of the distribution of nurses by Portuguese municipality will be carried out statically for the year 2002 - the youngest year for which there is the most complete and exhaustive statistical information at municipality level, considering the variables we want to study - and for the year 2010. This is the last year for which statistical information is available. In addition, in order to capture developments over the period considered (2002-2010), a dynamic econometric analysis will be carried out. This will include the variation in the variables between the two periods of time, in order to understand and quantify how the evolution of some of the explanatory variables over time affects the variation in the distribution of nurses in Portugal in the period in question.

Simultaneously with the OLS analysis, the Gini index will be presented, an index commonly used to quantify geographical inequality in the distribution of health care, including the distribution of health professionals, as described by Correia and Veiga (2010), who present a set of bibliographical references where the indicator is applied, as well as Toyabe (2009).

Both the OLS estimation and the calculation of the Gini index will be carried out using a set of statistical data collected from the *online* database of the National Statistics Institute (INE, 2011). The INE provides statistical information on the number of nurses per thousand inhabitants working in each of the 308 municipalities in mainland Portugal and the islands. The fact that information is available on the place of work of nurses is an added value for this work, since statistical information on health professionals is often only available by place of residence and not by place of work (Correia & Veiga, 2010). In fact, according to these authors who mention theories of location, those who offer goods and services tend to be close to those who seek them. Therefore, knowing the professional's place of work makes it possible to use an indicator that more accurately measures what is intended.

The data was processed using the *freeware* Greti econometric *software*, version 1.9.8[44] .

2.2.2. PRESENTATION, DESCRIPTION AND STATISTICAL ANALYSIS OF THE VARIABLES OF INTEREST

The variable to be analyzed is, as already mentioned, the distribution of the number of nurses per thousand inhabitants in the municipalities of mainland Portugal and the islands. This variable will be analyzed according to a set of selected variables that will explain the distribution of nursing professionals in the Portuguese municipalities. These variables are presented and described in the following table (Table 10). This table also shows the type of relationship expected between each of the explanatory variables and the one we wish to explain, as well as the strength of the expected relationship.

To identify the type of association between the explanatory variables and the explained variable, we used the notation (+) and (-) where (+) indicates a positive association and (-) a negative association. A positive association means that variations in the value of the

44 http://gretl.sourceforge.net/.

explanatory variable selected imply variations in the same direction in the explained variable. A negative association means that variations in the value of the selected explanatory variable imply variations in the opposite direction of the explained variable. To identify the strength of the expected associations, we used the notation (x) (xx) and (xxx). A greater number of x's indicates a greater expected strength in terms of the degree of association.

The selection of explanatory variables was based on the available literature (Correia & Veiga, 2010; Lin et al., 1997; Toyabe, 2009). Thus, given the existing literature, the following variables were selected which are believed to explain the geographical distribution of nurses across Portuguese municipalities: number of doctors per thousand inhabitants, number of beds per thousand inhabitants, existence (or not) of a central hospital, ageing index, total population, population aged 14 or under, masculinity index, old-age dependency index, mortality rate, number of nurses/doctors ratio and purchasing power index. Statistical values for these variables are available at county level for both 2002 and 2010. There is, however, one exception. For the purchasing power index, the last year for which statistical information is available is 2009. As this was considered an important variable in the analysis, it was decided to use the information for this point in time instead of abandoning the variable.

Table 10

Presentation and description of the variables under study, the type of association expected between the explanatory and explained variables and the respective strength of the expected relationship.

Variable	Description	Definition	Type of association expected	Strength of association expected
Nurse	Nurses per 1,000 inhabitants	Number of nurses per thousand inhabitants, by municipality where the workplace is located (explained variable)	n.a.	n.a.
Doctor	Doctors per 1,000 inhabitants	Number of doctors per thousand inhabitants, by place of residence (municipality)	(+)	(xxx)
Beds	Beds per 1,000 inhabitants	Number of beds per thousand inhabitants for an inpatient health facility (Health Centers and Hospitals)	(+)	(xx)
Population_T	Resident population	Number of people who live most of the year in the geographical location in question (municipality)	(+)	(x)
Population_0-14	Resident population aged 0-14	Number of people who live most of the year in the geographic location in question (municipality), and who are between the ages of 0 and 14, including	(+)	(x)
		Whether there is at least one hospital, public or		

		private, with all facilities in the municipality. Variable		
Hospital	Presence of a central hospital	*dummy*, which takes the value 1 if there is at least one public or private hospital with all facilities in the municipality; it takes the value 0 otherwise	(+)	(xxx)
Tx_mortality	Mortality rate	Number of deaths observed during a given period of time, usually a calendar year, relative to the average population of that period (variable expressed in number of deaths per 1,000 inhabitants)	(-)	(xx)
Ageing	ageing index	The ratio of the elderly population to the young population, usually defined as the quotient of the elderly population to the young population. number of people aged 65 and over and the number of people aged 0-14 (variable expressed per 100 people aged 0-14)	(+)	(x)
I_dependence	elderly dependency ratio	Ratio of the elderly population to the working-age population, usually defined as the quotient between the number of people aged 65 or over and the number of people aged 15-64 (variable expressed per 100 people aged 15-64)	(+)	(xx)
Lmasculinity	masculinity index (>65 years)	Ratio of male to female population (usually expressed per 100 women) over 65 years of age	(-)	(xx)
Longevity	longevity index	Ratio of the oldest-old population to the elderly population, usually defined as the quotient between the number of people aged 75 or over and the number of people aged 65 or over (usually expressed per 100 people aged 65 or over)	(+)	(xx)
NurseZmedic	Nurse/doctor ratio	Ratio between the number of nurses per thousand inhabitants and the number of doctors per thousand inhabitants in each municipality	(+)	(xxx)
IPC	purchasing power index	Purchasing Power Index *per capita*, by geographic location (in 2009, the closest year with statistical data available)	(+)	(xx)

Notes: n.a. means that this analysis does not apply to the variable; (+) means that a positive association is expected between the explanatory variable and the explained variable; (-) means that a negative association is expected between the explanatory variable and the explained variable; (x) (xx) and (xxx) indicates the strength of the association between the variables, with (x) representing a weaker association and (xx) a stronger relationship.

Source: Own elaboration based on the Integrated Metadata System of the National Statistics Institute, available at http://smi.ine.pt/.

Before presenting the selected variables and explaining the expected sign and strength of the association between each of the selected variables and the geographical distribution of nurses, it should be noted that the econometric analysis for 2002 and 2010 will use the logarithmized values of the variables. The aim is to make the values for each of the different municipalities more homogeneous, as these values can vary greatly from one municipality to another, and to present the results in terms of growth rates. In mathematical terms, the difference between two logarithmized values corresponds to an approximation between the growth rate of consecutive values of a variable. Only the *dummy* variable referring to the existence or not of a public or private central hospital will not be logarithmized. In economic terms, this approximation, in terms of growth rates, to the reading of the econometric results will make more sense than a reading in terms of the absolute values of the variables. For the econometric analysis of the variation between 2002 and 2010, the analysis will be carried out using the percentage growth rate of the variables. The choice of the percentage growth rate, rather than the logarithm, is due to the fact that the changes in the variables can be negative and therefore make it impossible to calculate the logarithm[45] . Below we will describe the variables to be used, why they are used and we will also explain their sign and the strength of the expected relationship.

The selection of the variable "number of doctors per thousand inhabitants" is important for the analysis because, as mentioned in Chapter I, the work of nurses, despite having some autonomy, is still very much dependent on doctors, particularly when it comes to prescribing medicines or complementary means of diagnosis (Lin et al., 1997; Wong et al., 2009 and Budge et al., 2003). It is also important not to forget the concept of skil-mix, where, as we have seen previously, the synergy of skills between doctors and nurses can be important in achieving a better quality of healthcare provision (Carr-Hill & Jenkins-Clarke, 2003; Blegen et al., 1998; Friesen, 1996). As such, it is hoped that where there are doctors, there will be nurses, so that this skill-mix can be enhanced. It is therefore expected that there will be a strong positive relationship between the geographical distribution of the number of doctors per thousand inhabitants and the geographical distribution of the number of nurses.

The variable number of beds per thousand inhabitants is expected to positively influence the distribution of nurses, although it is believed that the strength of the association is weak since nurses have increasingly differentiated roles and specialties (community nursing, medical-surgical nursing, rehabilitation nursing, child health/pediatric nursing, maternal health/obstetric nursing and, finally, mental health/psychiatric nursing) and the fact that there are beds does not necessarily mean that there are nurses, at least in the same proportion. As previously mentioned (Bloor & Maynard, 2003; Zurn et al., 2002), the ratio of inpatients to nurses is very difficult to predict, but it is suspected that in Portugal the ratio is high. In addition, there has been a downward trend in the number of beds and

45 This would generate situations of missing values and thus the abandonment of many observations in the econometric analysis of the evolution of the variables between 2002 and 2010.

hospitalization days, with an increase in outpatient surgeries (CNADCA, 2009). Thus, the number of beds per thousand inhabitants could have a positive influence on the geographical distribution of nurses in Portugal, albeit a weak one. Along the same lines, the presence of a central hospital is expected to explain the geographic distribution of nurses positively, but this time strongly, since central hospitals are the places of employment and therefore the reason for the geographic settlement of nurses par excellence.

The resident population per thousand inhabitants is also expected to positively influence the distribution of nurses (Henwood et al., 2009; Skillman et al., 2005), but with a weak strength of association since nurses are expected to be more present where there are more health care needs and not only where the resident population levels are higher.

As for the mortality rate, it is expected to show a negative association with the average strength of the geographical distribution of the professionals under study. The presence of nurses contributes, as mentioned by Aiken (1994), to a reduction in the mortality of patients and reduces the possibility of deaths due to complications caused by lack of care (Carr-Hill & Jenkins-Clarke, 2003; Blegen et al., 1998; Friesen, 1996). If the geographical distribution of nurses varies positively in a given municipality, it is expected that the variation in the mortality rate will be negative.

Finally, with regard to the purchasing power index, it was decided to check whether what Lin et al. (1997) described is happening in Portugal. According to the authors, nurses would tend to be located in places with greater purchasing power, namely urban areas. This aspect, also mentioned by Skillman et al. (2005) and Henwood et al. (2009), leads us to expect an average positive relationship between the purchasing power index and the location of nurses. Although it is not a fundamental factor in the location decision, it will be a factor of great importance in the analysis that will be carried out.

The other variables selected and shown in Table 10 were chosen by the author of this research paper. The purpose of selecting them was to see if any demographic characteristics related to the health and morbidity of the population influence the geographical distribution of nurses in Portugal.

It was decided to select a variable that measures the resident population aged between 0 and 14, since this age group traditionally requires special health care (health care related to vaccinations, monitoring congenital/acquired diseases and the high propensity to accidents), although to a lesser degree than the elderly. It is therefore expected that there will be a weak positive association between this variable and the geographical distribution of nurses.

Another of the variables selected is the population aging index. This indicator measures the ratio between the elderly population and the young population and is usually defined as the quotient between the number of people aged 65 or over and the number of people aged between 0 and 14. In other words, the higher this index is in a given municipality, the more elderly people there will be. It is expected that there will be a positive relationship, with a weak force, between the indicator and the distribution of nurses since, although there is a need for nurses in places with older people, it is not believed that the relationship will be so strongly positive since it is believed that political issues rather than demographic ones may have more weight in the distribution of nurses.

Other variables that may have some relevance in explaining the distribution of nursing professionals in Portugal include: the old-age dependency ratio, the longevity ratio, the masculinity ratio of people over 65 and the ratio of nurses to doctors in each municipality.

In the case of the elderly dependency index, it was hoped to verify the existence of a positive relationship, of average strength, between the variable and the geographical distribution of nurses, since very dependent elderly people have greater needs in terms of nursing care, particularly in nursing homes, retirement homes, day care centers and long-term care units. It was also decided to test the influence of the masculinity index for ages over 65, in order to see whether users of different genders and over 65 can influence the existence of a greater or lesser number of nurses in each municipality. It is believed that women seek health care more than men and therefore a negative association between the variables in question is to be expected. In the case of the longevity index, it is assumed that people who live longer also have this possibility due to the greater availability of nursing care, which is why a positive and medium-strength association is expected. Finally, it was decided to include the ratio of nurses to doctors in a given geographical location, using a simple calculation between the number of nurses per thousand inhabitants and the number of doctors. The aim is to see if the synergy between doctors and nurses influences the distribution of the number of nurses per thousand inhabitants. Given the concept of *skill-mix,* presented in the theoretical chapter, it is believed that if this ratio varies positively, the distribution of the number of nurses will vary in the same direction.

The statistical distribution of the values of the variables for 2002 and 2010 is shown below, both in absolute terms (Table 10) and in logarithm (Table 11). Note that the variable referring to the existence of a central hospital is not logarithmized because it is a variable that only takes on the value 1 (if there is a hospital in the geographical location) or 0 (when there isn't). The statistical distribution of the variation in each of the variables between 2002 and 2010 is also shown. The variation in the different variables between 2002 and 2010 is presented in absolute value and percentage for each variable, with the exception of the number of beds, where the variable is always presented in absolute value, and the existence (or not) of a central hospital, where, due to the binary nature of the variable, the option was made to maintain the value of the variable in 2010. To present these distributions, we chose to present a measure of central tendency (the mean) and some measures of variability - standard deviation, minimum and maximum value of the variable.

The indicators presented are calculated taking into account the observations (municipalities) for which statistical information is available. Whenever there are missing values, the observation is dropped.

Table 11

Statistical distribution of the absolute values of the selected variables for the years 2002 and 2010 and the respective variation between 2002-2010

Variable	2002				2010				Δ 2010-2002			
	Average	Standard Deviation	Minimum	Maximum	Average	Standard Deviation	Minimum	Maximum	Average	Standard Deviation	Minimum	Maximum
Nurse	2,2	2,8	0,0	20,9	4,0	3,5	0,0	26,5	1,8	1,5	-6,1	13,0
Medical	1,4	1,9	0,0	19,9	1,8	2,4	0,0	27,4	0,4	0,8	-5,3	7,5
Population	33.790,5	55.149,1	435,0	549.766,0	34.535,6	55.686,6	507,0	469.509,0	745,2	7.865,4	-80.257,0	74.502,0
Population_0-14	5.343,0	8.651,2	46,0	71.320,0	5.219,9	8.988,8	48,0	81.363,0	-123,1	1.204,6	-6.797,0	10.043,0
Mortality rate	13,0	4,0	5,0	26,5	12,9	4,6	5,4	29,2	-0,1	2,1	-7,4	8,0
I Ageing	154,6	80,8	33,6	523,3	175,2	87,2	34,4	538,7	20,6	29,3	-92,3	154,9
LDependence	33,0	12,8	12,8	83,9	33,8	11,4	12,1	78,5	0,8	4,2	-16,4	13,9
I Masculinity	94,6	4,6	76,6	120,4	71,7	7,6	37,9	96,0	-23,0	5,4	-44,0	-8,0

Beds	1,4	2,5	0,0	16,8	1,1	2,9	0,0	20,9	-0,4	1,7	-15,0	9,3
Hospital	0,3	0,5	0,0	1,0	0,3	0,5	0,0	1,0	-	-	-	-
LLongevity	44,0	3,8	30,7	54,6	50,8	5,5	35,7	65,8	6,8	3,6	-10,7	19,2
Nurse/doctor	1,9	1,8	0,0	14,0	3,1	3,1	0,0	28,0	1,2	2,7	-8,9	22,8
IPC	69,2	26,8	36,2	220,2	75,7	24,0	47,4	232,5	6,4	9,4	-35,2	37,3

Source: Own calculations based on INE information

Table 12

Statistical distribution of the yogarithmized values of the selected variables for the years 2002 and 2010 and their growth rate between 2000 and 2010

Variable	2002				2010				Δ 2010-2002			
	Average	Standard Deviation	Minimum	Maximum	Average	Standard Deviation	Minimum	Maximum	Average	Standard Deviation	Minimum	Maximum
Nurse	0,35	0,86	-2,30	3,04	1,15	0,65	-1,61	3,28	1,70	2,56	-1,00	26,00
Medical	0,00	0,81	-2,30	2,99	0,27	0,77	-2,30	3,31	0,42	0,98	-1,00	14,00
Population	9,75	1,10	6,08	13,22	9,74	1,14	6,23	13,06	0,00	0,09	-0,19	0,41
Population_0-14	7,82	1,20	3,83	11,17	7,72	1,27	3,87	11,31	-0,08	0,15	-0,33	0,57
Mortality rate	2,52	0,31	1,61	3,28	2,49	0,35	1,69	3,37	-0,01	0,15	-0,47	0,56
I Ageing	4,92	0,50	3,51	6,26	5,06	0,47	3,54	6,29	0,18	0,33	-0,73	3,14
LDependence	3,42	0,38	2,55	4,43	3,47	0,34	2,49	4,36	0,06	0,17	-0,58	0,90
I Masculinity	4,55	0,05	4,34	4,79	4,27	0,11	3,63	4,56	-0,24	0,06	-0,51	-0,08
Qamas	0,70	0,88	-2,30	2,82	1,05	0,95	-1,20	3,04	-0,41	1,71	-15,00	9,30
Longevity	3,78	0,09	3,42	4,00	3,92	0,11	3,58	4,19	0,15	0,08	-0,20	0,63
Nurse/doctor	0,35	0,81	-1,90	2,64	0,88	0,70	-1,50	3,33	1,17	2,57	-1,00	33,18
IPQ	4,18	0,33	3,59	5,39	4,29	0,27	3,86	5,45	0,12	0,14	-0,27	0,59

Notes: For Δ 2010-2002 the values should be understood as the percentage growth rates read in decimal places. For beds, the absolute value of the change.

Source: Own calculations based on INE information

As we've seen in previous sections, the number of nurses per thousand inhabitants rose sharply between 2002 and 2010, with some municipalities having as many as 26.5 nurses per thousand inhabitants in 2010, while others had no nurses at all. It should be noted that between 2002 and 2010, there were municipalities with a negative variation in the number of nurses per thousand inhabitants (-6.1 nurses per thousand inhabitants) and others with a sharp increase (13 nurses per thousand inhabitants). In average terms, there was an increase of 1.8 nurses per thousand inhabitants in Portuguese municipalities between 2002 and 2010.

With regard to the total resident population, there was an average upward trend. Attention should be drawn to the fact that there are municipalities with a large variation in the number of inhabitants over the period analyzed, which indicates that there has been a considerable migration of the population from their municipalities of residence. Although the analysis is not presented here, it is believed that this movement is due to the migration of the population between rural and more urban municipalities. As for the resident population aged 14 and under, there has been a negative variation in the average values, a clear reflection of the inversion trend of the Portuguese age pyramid in recent years, something that should be a cause for concern.

Looking at the mortality rate figures in the table showing the distribution of the indicator in absolute value, it should be noted that they have remained practically unchanged. The same is true of the old-age dependency ratio. Antagonistic changes can be seen in the variables relating to the ageing index and the masculinity index calculated for the population aged over 65. For the first indicator, there was an upward trend (which, as with the resident population aged between 0 and 14, confirms the upward trend of the Portuguese age pyramid). For the second indicator, the masculinity index, there has been a downward trend in the percentage of men over 65 compared to the number of women of the same age, i.e. there has been a large decrease in the proportion of men over 65 compared to the number of women (on average, by municipality, there has been a 23% decrease in the index), which confirms the common wisdom that there is a higher percentage of women in this age group.

As for the number of doctors per thousand inhabitants, as we have seen in previous sections, there is also an upward trend in this indicator. On average, the number of doctors per thousand inhabitants grew by 0.4 per municipality. In 2010, there was at least one municipality with 27.4 doctors per thousand inhabitants and another with no doctors at all. These figures, like those for the number of nurses, reveal the existence of major asymmetries between Portuguese municipalities. In terms of the ratio of nurses to doctors[46] , there is a tendency for the average values to increase (from 1.9 nurses per doctor per municipality on average in 2002, to 3.1 in 2010, corresponding to an average increase of 1.2 nurses per doctor on average). This increase reflects the higher average growth in the number of nurses than in the number of doctors, perhaps due to an increase in the supply of trained nursing professionals (OECD, 2011b; DGES, 2012) and possibly to a readjustment of the skills of each of these professionals (*skill-mix*).

As for the variable referring to the presence of a central hospital, its variation was not analyzed since there were no major variations, however, the number of beds per thousand inhabitants shows a downward trend. This is explained by the introduction of policies to increase the number of outpatient surgeries/procedures (CNADCA, 2009), hence the downward trend in the number of beds. However, there are a large number of missing values in the number of beds per thousand inhabitants variable. These omitted values lead to the abandonment of many observations (municipalities), so that what could *a priori* be an important variable for studying the geographical distribution of the number of nurses per thousand inhabitants can present problems of application in the OLS model.

Finally, with regard to the purchasing power index, the distribution of statistical values shows a tendency for the average values to increase, which may represent an increase in the quality of life of citizens. With regard to purchasing power asymmetries between 2002 and 2010, the minimum and maximum values increased in the same proportion, but there is still a huge gap between the richest and poorest municipalities, as shown, for example, in the OECD report entitled "*Divided we stand: why inequality keeps rising",* in which Portugal is presented as the OECD country with the greatest inequalities between rich and poor from the 1980s until 2008 (OECD, 2011d).

2.2.3. Measuring inequality in the distribution of nurses in Portugal: the Gini index

The Gini index, as already mentioned, is a coefficient widely used to measure the distributive equity of certain population factors, and is particularly used in the health sector, for example in Correia and Veiga (2010)[47] and Toyabe (2009). Both studies deal with the application of the indicator to analyze the geographical distribution of doctors. Munga and

46 It should be remembered that the indicator was calculated by the author for this research work on the basis of the statistical data available for nurses and doctors per 1,000 inhabitants.

47 The authors present an extensive list of bibliographical references where the Gini index has been applied to analyze the phenomenon of equity in the distribution of health resources.

Maestad (2009) also present a study to analyze the inequality of the distribution of various health professionals.

The Gini coefficient has values between 0 and 1, and the closer the value is to 0, the greater the distributional equity. Conversely, the closer the index value is to 1, the more unequal the distribution of the variable under analysis. In this research, using the Greti econometric *software*, the Gini index is calculated using the following formula (Cottrell & Lucchetti, 2012):

$$G = \frac{2\sum_{i=1}^{n} iy_i}{n\sum_{i=1}^{n} y_i} - \frac{n+1}{n} \quad (1)$$

Where, G is the Gini index, i corresponds to a given municipality i, n is the number of observations (municipalities) and y_i is the value of the variable under analysis in municipality i.

By applying the formula to the variables number of nurses and doctors per thousand inhabitants, total resident population and purchasing power index, the values shown in Table 13 were obtained for 2002 and 2010. The same table also shows the values for the coefficient of variation for the same indicators and for the same two periods of time. The coefficient of variation describes the dispersion of the variable as a percentage, i.e. it describes how the variable disperses around the average value without this measure being affected by the unit of measurement of the variable. In statistical terms, the coefficient of variation is calculated as the ratio between the standard deviation and the mean value of the variable. In terms of analysis, the higher the coefficient of variation, the greater the percentage dispersion of the variable.

Table 13

Gini index and coefficients of variation for 2002 and 2010

Year	Nurses		Doctors		Total population		Purchasing power index	
	Gini index	Coefficient of variation	Gini index	Coefficient of variation	Gini index	Coefficient of variation	Gini index	Coefficient of variation
2002	0,505	1,271	0,471	1,308	0,604	1,632	0,197	0,388
2010	0,380	0,880	0,452	1,327	0,612	1,612	0,158	0,317

Source: Own elaboration based on INE data

Graphically, the value of the Gini index can be visualized using the Lorenz curve (shown in red in the figures below). The Lorenz curve represents the proportion of the total value of the variable (vertical axis) that is obtained by the cumulative sum of the values observed for the municipalities (starting from the one with the lowest value to the one with the highest value) and which are represented on the horizontal axis. The bisector of the graph (45° line) represents a situation of perfect equality in the distribution of the variable under study (shown in blue in the figures below). In view of the above, the value of the Gini index corresponds to the ratio between the area between the 45° line and the Lorenz curve and the total area below the 45° line (Munga & Maestad, 2009).

Figures 15 and 16 show the Lorenz curves for the different indicators for 2002 and 2010, respectively.

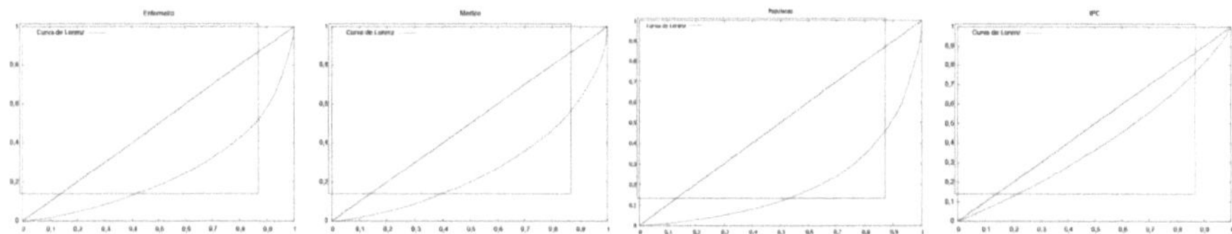

Figure 15: Lorenz curves for 2002

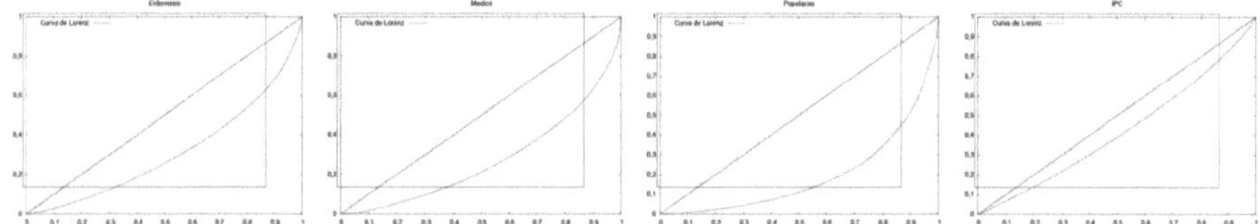

Figure 16: Lorenz curves for 2010

As can be seen in table 13, the Gini coefficient calculated for the distribution of the number of nurses in Portugal in 2002 and 2010 fell sharply from 0.505 to 0.380, which means that there is a trend towards greater equity in the distribution of these professionals across the country. It should also be noted that there was also a notable decrease in the coefficient of variation from 2002 to 2010, i.e. a decrease in the average deviation of the number of nurses in relation to the national average. Graphical analysis shows this positive trend, with the Lorenz curve approaching the 45 degree line (figures 15 and 16). In terms of comparison, it can be seen that the Gini index also decreased for the geographical distribution of the number of doctors, but to a much lesser extent (from 0.471 to 0.452) than for nurses, so that the graphical analysis of the Lorenz curve shows almost no differences. The same trend was no longer seen for the total resident population, even showing a worsening of the distributive equity of the population in that there was an increase in the gini index from 0.604 in 2002 to 0.612 in 2010, which confirms data that indicates a worsening of the urban/rural divide. The indicator measuring purchasing power is the one with the highest levels of equity (approximately 0.2 in 2002 and 0.16 in 2010) since the value is closer to zero and the Lorenz curve is closer to the bisector of the corresponding graph (Figure 15 and 16). Analysis of the values calculated for the coefficient of variation confirms the analysis carried out earlier.

Given that there is some inequality in the distribution of the number of nurses per municipality in Portugal, and despite the fact that there was a tendency for this inequality to diminish between 2002 and 2010, an attempt will be made to identify and quantify the determinants that explain this inequality.

2.2.4. DETERMINANTS OF THE DISTRIBUTION OF NURSES IN PORTUGAL: STATIC OLS MODEL

Static OLS will be applied to identify and quantify the determinants of the geographical distribution of nurses in Portugal in a given year, in particular[48] . The analysis will be carried out for 2002 and then for 2010. In the statistical models applied to each of these years, the dependent variable will be the logarithm of nurses per thousand inhabitants. The models differ in the explanatory variables they use. In total, the results for 7 different models will be presented.

Models 1 and 2 use all the variables considered relevant in order to understand which ones influence the geographical distribution of nurses and how they explain the variation in the distribution of the number of nurses per thousand inhabitants. As the indicator of the ratio between the number of nurses and doctors per thousand inhabitants is calculated using the variables number of nurses per thousand inhabitants and number of doctors per thousand inhabitants, the three variables cannot be used together in the same model given the problems of perfect multicollinearity. Therefore, model 1 uses the variable number of doctors per thousand inhabitants and model 2 uses the ratio of nurses to doctors as the explanatory variable.

Model 3 presents, as explanatory variables, those which may be representative of the presence of specific infrastructures (beds and central hospital) and specialized personnel (doctors) and which, in this way, can explain the number of nurses in a given municipality. Model 4 aims to test whether the geographical distribution of the number of nurses is influenced by the number of inhabitants (total and young inhabitants) in a given municipality. Model 5 aims to see if the number of nurses could be influenced by the existence of a population traditionally more in need of care, such as the elderly or groups

48 The distinction between static and dynamic models follows the distinction made by Correia & Veiga (2010) and may not conform to any other type of technical distinction between the two models.

with lower financial resources. Model 5 will therefore present the mortality rate and the indices of old-age dependency, ageing, longevity, masculinity and purchasing power as explanatory variables. Model 6 will estimate the influence of all the variables under analysis with the exception of the number of beds and the presence of a central hospital. In this model, the ratio of nurses to doctors will be used instead of the number of doctors per thousand inhabitants.

Finally, model 7 will use, as explanatory variables, the variables with the highest statistically significant correlation coefficient[49] between their logarithmic value and the number of nurses per thousand inhabitants, in logarithm. The correlation coefficient between the logarithm of the values of each of the explanatory variables and the logarithm of the number of nurses per thousand inhabitants is shown in Table 14. The table shows the significance level for which the correlation coefficient is statistically significant, as well as the number of observations (in brackets) used to calculate the coefficient for each pair of variables. Variables for which the correlation coefficient is not statistically significant at at least a 10% significance level are shaded.

Table 14

Correlation coefficient between each of the explanatory variables and the number of nurses per thousand inhabitants in 2002 and 2010 and considering the variation of the variables between 2002-2010.

Time	Medical	Population	Population_0-14	Tx_mortality	I_Aging	I_Dependence	I_Masculinity	Beds	I_Longevity	Nurse/doctor	IPC	Hospital
2002	0,5369 * (303)	0,2453 * (306)	0,2144 * (306)	-0,0153 (306)	0,0188 (306)	-0,0294 (306)	-0,1294 ** (306)	0,7254 * (126)	-0,0029 (306)	0,5318 * (306)	0,3837 * (306)	0,3106 * (306)
2010	0,5238 * (304)	0,2969 * (307)	0,2648 * (307)	-0,0080 (307)	-0,0314 (307)	-0,0881 (307)	-0,1873 * (307)	0,7565 * (63)	-0,0975 *** (307)	0,3600 * (307)	0,2926 * (307)	0,2807 * (307)
Δ 2010-2002	0,0799 (303)	-0,0078 (306)	-0,1058 *** (306)	0,0032 (306)	0,0596 (306)	-0,0428 (306)	-0,2505 * (306)	-0,0098 (253)	0,0896 (306)	0,7526 * (306)	0,2271 * (306)	0,1439 ** (306)

Notes: The correlation coefficient was calculated for the logarithmized values of the variables; The number of observations used to calculate the correlation coefficient is shown in parentheses; * indicates that the value is statistically significant at a significance

49 *Pearson*'s correlation coefficient is the most powerful coefficient and can only be used with quantitative variables. It is a parametric correlation coefficient. This type of correlation coefficient involves carrying out a hypothesis test in which the null hypothesis states that the correlation between the variables is null (Martinez & Aristides, 2010).

level of 1%; ** indicates that the value is statistically significant at a significance level of 5% and *** means that the value is statistically significant at a significance level of 10%.

Source: Own elaboration based on INE data

It can be seen that in the two time periods (first two lines) there is a statistically significant correlation, at a significance level of 1%, between the number of nurses per thousand inhabitants (in logarithm) and the variables corresponding to the number of doctors per thousand inhabitants and the ratio of nurses to doctors, for the same population measure. However, for the period between 2002 and 2010, the variation in the number of doctors is no longer statistically correlated with the variation in the number of nurses, while the ratio of nurses to doctors increases its strength of relationship.

Another variable that maintains statistically significant correlation levels for the time periods considered is the variable measuring the youth population (population aged between 0 and 14). The correlation coefficient obtained for the total population variable is also statistically significant for 2002 and 2010, but the variation in the population between these two time points does not seem to be statistically correlated with the variation in the number of nurses per thousand inhabitants. The existence, or not, of a hospital in the municipality, as well as the number of inpatient beds, are variables that are also highly correlated with the number of nurses per thousand inhabitants. It should be noted, however, that the use of the variable corresponding to the number of beds implies the loss of many observations (and consequent degrees of freedom in the estimation) since the information for many Portuguese municipalities is missing.

Also noteworthy is the fact that the purchasing power index variable shows interesting correlation values, at a significance level of 1%, in the three periods considered.

It should be noted that the mortality rate, old-age dependency ratio, ageing index and longevity index generally do not show statistically significant correlation coefficients between their values and the number of nurses per thousand inhabitants.

In view of the above, we chose to present the total and youth populations, the purchasing power index, the existence (or not) of a hospital, the masculinity index and the ratio of nurses to doctors as explanatory variables in model 7.

Possible multicollinearity problems (existence of non-zero covariance between the explanatory variables selected to estimate the seven different models) were checked for all the models. The variance inflation factors (*VIF)* used (Cottrell & Lucchetti, 2012) did not indicate serious problems of multicollinearity between the explanatory variables, so the choice of variables for each of the models did not present any technical problems for the estimation of the models using the OLS methodology or for the interpretation of the estimated coefficients.

Table 15 shows the results of the estimation of the 7 models presented above for the year 2002, so that we can see which variables influence the motivation for the distribution of the number of nurses per thousand inhabitants in this period. The aim is also to understand the extent to which these variables influence the variable we are trying to explain. The table shows the estimated coefficients for the variables selected in each of the different models proposed, as well as their standard deviation (in brackets) and the level of statistical significance of each estimated coefficient.

Table 15

Results of the static OLS models for 2002

Variables	Model 1	Model 2	Model 3	Model 4	Model 5	Model 6	Model 7
Medical	0,286 ***	---	0,359 ***	---	---	-	---
	(0,105)		(0,072)				
Population	-1,716	-1,553	---	1,107	---	-2,040	0,682 ***
	(3,178)	(3,045)		(0,344)		(1,711)	(0,243)
Population_0-14	1,732	1,682	---	-0,939	---	2,199	-0,623 ***
	(3,163)	(3,040)		(0,300)		(1,725)	(0,214)
Tx_Mortality	0,684 *	0,221	---	---	0,715 **	0,369	---
	(0,366)	(0,307)			(0,340)	(0,272)	
I_Aging	1,878	1,046	---	---	0,380	2,281	---
	(2,723)	(2,645)			(0,434)	(1,520)	
I_Dependence	-1,662	-0,293	---	---	-0,999	-2,086 *	---
	(2,191)	(2,118)			(0,657)	(1,227)	
I_Masculinity	0,900	0,228	---	---	-2,228 **	-1,205	-1,498 *
	(1,160)	(0,873)			(1,002)	(0,862)	(0,876)
Beds	0,562 ***	0,364 ***	0,544 ***	---	---	---	---
	(0,080)	(0,088)	(0,063)				
I_Longevity	-1,941 ***	0,129	---	---	1,970 **	1,902 ***	---
	(0,740)	(0,802)			-0,933	(0,658)	
Nurse/doctor	---	0,520 ***	---	---	---	0,744 ***	0,744 ***
		(0,104)				(0,041)	(0,046)
IPC	0,250	1,161 ***	---	---	1,230 ***	1,424 ***	1,354 ***
	(0,252)	(0,238)			(0,194)	(0,142)	(0,145)
Hospital	0,055	0,061	0,028	0,454	---	---	0,177 **
	(0,101)	(0,084)	(0,090)	(0,129)			(0,074)

Constant	0,353	-9,013 *	0,284 ***	3,250 ***	-2,346	-9,861 **	-0,581
	(6,580)	(4,607)	(0,070)	(1,107)	5,668	(4,951)	(4,249)
Observations	126	126	126	306	306	306	306
Adjusted R2	0,652	0,766	0,634	0,135	0,197	0,650	0,635
F-test	32,626 ***	40,516 ***	76,817 ***	11,577 ***	9,946 ***	65,090 ***	70,931 ***

Notes: Standard deviation values are shown in brackets; * indicates that the coefficient is statistically significant at a significance level of 10%; ** indicates that the coefficient is statistically significant at a significance level of 5% and *** means that the coefficient is statistically significant at a significance level of 1%; - indicates that the variable in question was not used in the estimation.

It should be noted that the models are estimated based on *cross-section* data - the data for each of the variables is presented per observation (municipality) at a single point in time - which may bring with it problems of heteroscedasticity - the variance of the error term may not be constant between municipalities (Gujarati, 2004) and so the variance of the estimated coefficients is not guaranteed to be minimal. Heteroscedasticity problems were tested for each model and corrected using MacKinnon and White's methodology for calculating consistent robust standard errors in *cross-sectional* data (Cottrell & Lucchetti, 2012; Davidson & MacKinnon, 2003). In this way, all the results for the estimated models (for 2002, presented above, 2010 and for the variation between 2002 and 2010, presented below) present robust standard errors that correct the heteroscedasticity problems.

All seven models estimated in Table 15 have an F-statistic, which tests the joint significance of the selected explanatory variables, which is statistically significant at a 1% significance level. Thus, all the models presented bring together a set of variables that simultaneously explain the distribution of nurses by municipality in Portugal in 2002.

However, some of the models are more explanatory of the variable under analysis - the distribution of nurses. Models 4 and 5 show values for the adjusted coefficient of determination (adjusted[50]) of less than 20% (13.5% in model 4 and 19.7% in model 5). This indicates that the variation in the variables included in both models explains only 13.5% and 19.7%, respectively, of the variation in the distribution of the number of nurses per 1,000 inhabitants in Portugal in 2002. The models therefore seem to have little explanatory value. This suggests that trying to explain the distribution of the number of nurses per 1,000 inhabitants in Portuguese municipalities using demographic variables is

50 Note that the adjusted coefficient of determination is presented instead of the coefficient of determination so that its value is adjusted to the degrees of freedom of each model and is not sensitive to the number of explanatory variables included in it.

not at all sufficient to explain this distribution. The remaining models have adjusted determination coefficients of over 63%. Model 2 (which includes all the variables considered in this study with the exception of the number of doctors per 1,000 inhabitants for the reasons explained) has an explanatory power of around 77% for the percentage variation in the number of nurses per 1,000 inhabitants between Portuguese municipalities in 2002. In other words, the percentage variation in the variables considered explains around 77% of the percentage variation in the distribution of nurses per municipality.

It should be noted, however, that only 126 municipalities are considered for models 1 and 2. The lack of information for the remaining municipalities meant that the figure for the number of beds was omitted and therefore not taken into account in the analysis. For the remaining models, because the number of beds variable was not taken into account, 306 Portuguese counties were used in the analysis.

In model 2, estimated for 126 municipalities and the one whose included variables have the greatest explanatory power, only 3 variables show individual statistical significance. The number of beds observed in the municipality, the ratio of nurses to doctors in the municipality and the purchasing power index. A 1% variation in the number of beds between municipalities in 2002 meant that the number of nurses per 1,000 inhabitants varied in the same direction by around 0.36%. With 99% certainty, it is estimated that, in 2002, doubling the number of beds in a municipality would increase the number of nurses per 1,000 inhabitants by 1/3 in that municipality. It should be noted that in this model, as is the case for all models in which the existence (or not) of a central hospital is taken into account (with the exception of model 7), the *dummy* variable that measures this fact, despite always having a positive estimator, is statistically non-significant. More than the existence or not of a hospital in the municipality, the number of beds seems to be fundamental in determining the distribution of nurses. These results suggest that other institutions, whether included in the SNS or not, can determine the number of nurses. As long as there are "beds" to receive patients, there is a need for nurses.

Still analyzing model 2, we see that the purchasing power index seems to have had a more substantial effect than the number of beds in 2002. At a significance level of 1%, it can be seen that in 2002, if the purchasing power of a municipality was 1% higher in a given municipality, this would mean that the number of nurses per thousand inhabitants in that municipality would be around 1.16% higher. The purchasing power of the population is therefore a fundamental aspect in explaining the distribution of the number of nurses in Portugal in 2002 - they would tend to be located in places with higher purchasing power, in line with the reference literature (Lin et al., 1997; Skillman et al., 2005 and Henwood et al., 2009). In other words, places that can provide them with greater purchasing power and also with greater capacity to take advantage of their services, particularly in the private sector. The importance of this variable is confirmed by looking at the results for the other models. Its value is always positive and statistically significant at a 1% significance level. The only model in which this is not the case is the model that replaces the ratio of nurses to doctors with the variable measuring the number of doctors per 1,000 inhabitants (model 1). In this model, the variable remains positive but loses "explanatory power" and statistical significance.

Note that model 2 shows the number of nurses per doctor in a given municipality as one of the explanatory variables, whereas model 1 shows the number of doctors per thousand inhabitants instead. What the results of model 2 (and also those of models 6 and 7) show, with 99% certainty, is that whenever the ratio of nurses to doctors increases by 1% (indicating an increase in the autonomy of nursing activity in relation to medical activity) the number of nurses in a given municipality increases by 0.52% (almost 0.75% in models 6 and 7). The autonomy of nurses in relation to doctors thus seems to have been an important explanatory factor for the distribution of nurses in Portuguese municipalities in 2002. But also the number of doctors per thousand inhabitants. The results of model 1 show, also with 99% certainty, that whenever the number of doctors per thousand inhabitants increased in a municipality by 1% compared to the other municipalities, the number of nurses increased by around 0.29%. The distribution of nurses depends positively on the distribution of the number of doctors, but is determined even more strongly by the autonomy of nursing activity in relation to medical activity. This conclusion may reinforce the conclusion drawn with regard to the variables related to the number of beds and the existence of a central hospital. Correia and Veiga (2010) verified the importance of the existence of a central hospital in explaining the distribution of doctors in Portugal. In addition, the central hospital is a determining factor in attracting doctors to a municipality. These imply the need for more nurses. The results of model 3 reinforce this conclusion. However, whenever nursing activity can be carried out more autonomously, this can determine the distribution of nurses per municipality very positively.

In model 7, as expected given the statistically significant correlation between the explanatory variables included in the model, all the variables are individually statistically significant. In 2002, the existence of a central hospital explained a positive difference of almost 0.18% in the number of nurses per municipality. If the ratio of nurses to doctors increased by 1% in a given municipality, the number of nurses per thousand inhabitants would also be higher by almost 0.75%. If that municipality had a 1% higher purchasing power, all other things being equal, the number of nurses in that municipality would be 1.35% higher, which is quite significant, especially when compared to the previous variables.

These figures confirm conclusions already drawn for other models, but the novelty of model 7 is now related to the statistical importance assumed by the variables that try to "capture" the importance of population size. A 1% increase in the total population of a Portuguese municipality would increase the number of nurses in that municipality by around 0.68%, however, if only the population aged 14 or under is analyzed, the opposite effect seems to occur. In 2002, a 1% increase in the young population (0-14 years) would mean a 0.65% decrease in the number of nurses, contrary to what would be expected given the needs of this type of population (as described in previous sections). This joint result may indicate that the increase in the number of nurses in a municipality is more related to another type of population - an older population. In fact, in model 5, which combines variables that only try to express some demographic characteristics of the population, despite their weak explanatory power, it can be seen that a 1% increase in the population's longevity index increased the number of nurses per thousand inhabitants in that municipality by 1.97%. Increases in the mortality rate of 1% (normal increases in older populations) also increased the number of nurses per municipality by around 0.72%.

Another interesting fact to analyze is the negative influence that, in 2002, increases in the masculinity index had on the distribution of nurses by municipality (models 5 and 7). Older women are the ones who traditionally seek health care the most and also live the longest, and these results seem to demonstrate this.

For 2010, the estimated results are shown in the following table. This table shows the estimated results for the same seven models mentioned above. The results will be analyzed for 2010 in particular, taking into account the changes compared to 2002.

Table 16

Results of the static OLS models for 2010

Variables	Model 1	Model 2	Model 3	Model 4	Model 5	Model 6	Model 7
Medical	0,228 ** (0,098)	---	0,364 *** (0,053)	-	-	---	---
Population	0,400 (0,516)	0,840 ** (0,359)	---	1,023 *** (0,251)	-	0,929 *** (0,282)	1,114 *** (0,191)

Population_0-14	-0,356	-0,650 *		-0,817 ***		-0,705 **	0,935 ***
	(0,486)	(0,358)		(0,208)		(0,282)	(0,168)
Tx_Mortality	0,494	0,708 **	---	-	0,351 *	0,411 **	---
	(0,329)	(0,311)			(0,187)	(0,172)	
I_Aging	1,192 **	1,173 ***	---	-	2,027 ***	0,951 ***	---
	(0,451)	(0,438)			(0,366)	(0,313)	
MDependence	-2,020 ***	-2,028 ***	---	-	-3,053 ***	-1,772 ***	---
	(0,602)	(0,603)			(0,544)	(0,455)	
I_Masculinity	-0,221	-0,272			-0,930 ***	-0,406	-0,914 ***
	(0,518)	(0,466)			(0,348)	(0,308)	(0,276)
Beds	0,300 ***	0,262 ***	0,367 ***				
	(0,062)	(0,077)	(0,052)				
I_Longevity	0,330	0,018	---	-	-	0,726	---
	(0,942)	(1,036)				(0,509)	
Nurse/doctor	---	0,328 ***	---	-	-	0,527 ***	0,559 ***
		(0,120)				(0,058)	(0,058)
IPC	0,572 **	1,038 ***	---	-	1,278 ***	1,354 ***	1,208 ***
	(0,240)	(0,353)			(0,180)	(0,194)	(0,168)
Hospital	0,034	0,096	-0,077	0,224 **	-	---	0,145 **
	(0,141)	(0,133)	(0,097)	(0,101)			(0,068)
Constant	-3,181	-6,463	1,007 ***	-2,589 ***	-3,168	-9,547 ***	-4,310 ***
	(4,383)	(4,314)	(0,077)	(0,901)	(3,193)	(2,695)	(1,459)
Observations	62	63	62	307	307	307	307
Adjusted R2	0,747	0,750	0,732	0,146	0,252	0,530	0,507
F-test	52,020 ***	23,541 ***	101,697 ***	12,953 ***	13,168 ***	32,300 ***	41,559 ***

Notes: Standard deviation values are shown in brackets; * indicates that the coefficient is statistically significant at a 10% significance level;

** indicates that the coefficient is statistically significant at a significance level of 5% and *** means that the coefficient is statistically significant at a significance level of 1%; - indicates that the variable in question was not used in the estimation.

For 2010, the models indicate a slightly different scenario to the one observed for 2002.

From 2002 to 2010, there was an increase in the number of explanatory variables with individual statistical significance. As was the case in 2002, in 2010 all seven estimated models showed a statistically significant F-test value at a 1% significance level. Thus, all the models presented seem to bring together a set of variables that simultaneously explain the distribution of nurses by municipality in Portugal in 2010, with a 99% degree of certainty. In 2010, there was also an increase in the degree of explanation of the variation in the distribution of nurses in Portugal, in most models, to the extent that there was an increase in the adjusted level compared to 2002, with the exception of models 3 and 6. In 2010, models 1, 2 and 3 had a high degree of explanation (between 73 and 75%) for the distribution of nurses. It should be noted, however, that the number of observations (63 and 62) was lower due to the existence of missing values in the number of beds variable for 2010.

If we look at models 4 and 5, we can see that they have values for the adjusted coefficient of determination of 14.6% and 25.2% respectively, the latter having increased considerably compared to 2002. As model 5 essentially contains variables related to population health factors, this increase in explanatory power may be due to the greater importance given to these factors by nurse distribution policies. It seems that greater importance is being given to factors such as the ageing index and the old-age dependency index in the distribution of nurses, and the expansion of the long-term care network may have contributed to this paradigm shift. Model 5 shows particularly interesting results for the dependency ratio and the aging ratio, which appear to have different effects on the distribution of nurses, at county level, for 2010 and for a significance level of 1%. The results of model 5 show, with 99% certainty, that whenever the dependency ratio increases in a municipality by 1% compared to the other municipalities, the number of nurses decreases by around 3%. On the other hand, whenever the ageing index increases by 1%, the number of nurses in these municipalities will increase by around 2%. The same is true of models 1 and 2, although to a lesser extent. This seems to indicate that there is a tendency for nurses to be located in areas with a higher concentration of elderly people, namely in nursing homes and long-term care facilities. The inverse proportionality between the number of nurses and the dependency index can be explained by the fact that the increase in these professionals in 2010 in the above-mentioned contexts contributed to a decrease in dependency, hence the antagonistic relationship with the number of nurses.

Also noteworthy is the fact that, in model 3, the three variables considered (doctor per thousand inhabitants, beds per thousand inhabitants and presence of a central hospital) explain approximately 73% of the variation in the number of nurses in Portugal, which means that, in 2010, the presence of nurses was very dependent on these variables. This result is very important because, in addition, only the variable measuring the presence of a central hospital is not statistically significant. The model shows that every 1% increase in the number of doctors per thousand inhabitants implies a 0.64% increase in the number of nurses, which is in line with the literature consulted and similar to that found for 2002. A similar situation can be seen with the number of beds per thousand inhabitants, although there is a reduction in magnitude compared to 2002. According to model 4, every 1% increase in the presence of a central hospital in the municipalities implies a 0.22% increase in the number of nurses. The presence of a central hospital is an important and statistically significant variable in explaining the distribution of the number of nurses, despite the trend towards a reduction in the number of these professionals in some hospitals as there are closures of certain services, which can be fundamental in positively influencing the number of nurses in a given geographical location.

Another interesting situation is the purchasing power index. According to model 6, it can be said with 99% certainty that each 1% increase in the purchasing power index in each municipality will imply an increase in the number of nurses of around 1.35%. Although this is in line with 2002, it reinforces the conclusion that purchasing power has a great deal of influence on the distribution of nurses at county level in Portugal. This factor is even more interesting when coupled with the previous improvement in the distributive equity of these professionals between 2002 and 2010 (Gini coefficient closer to zero in 2010 than in 2002) and the fact that factors related to the health status of the population (model 5) had a growing influence on the distribution of nurses in 2010. In other words, regardless of the fact that there may have been a readjustment in the policies for distributing these professionals, purchasing power continues to be very influential, even more so than the number of doctors per municipality, whose increase of 1% implies an increase in the number of nurses of 0.36% (according to model 3 and for a significance level of 1%).

Looking only at model 7, it can be said, at a significance level of 1%, that, contrary to what happened in 2002, increases of 1% in the total population and in the population aged 14 and under, imply an increase in the number of nurses of 1.11 and 0.95%, respectively. However, it should be noted that in the other models in which the variable was used (models 1, 2, 4 and 6) the relationship was always negative, so there may not have been a change compared to 2002. In other words, this type of population may have difficulties accessing these professionals, despite their characteristics.

It is also important to note the greater individual statistical significance of the mortality rate in 2010 compared to 2002, where, according to model 6, each 1% increase in the mortality rate per municipality in Portugal corresponds to an increase of around 0.41% in the number of nurses in that municipality. This seems to contradict the literature consulted (Meadows et al., 2000; Aiken et al., 2003 and Bigbee, 2008), which argues that an increase in the number of nurses is related to a decrease in the mortality rate. However, it is believed that in this static model, an increase in the number of nurses in a given municipality is related to an increase in mortality, with the aim of having the opposite effect in the medium and long term, so this conclusion can only be drawn in the dynamic model. In model 5, it can be seen that the masculinity index, as in 2002, maintains a negative correlation with the number of nurses. It can be said with 99% certainty that for every 1% increase in the masculinity index, the number of nurses decreases by 0.93%, which despite being a smaller difference than in 2002, maintains the tendency for female users to make greater use of the services provided by nurses.

2.2.5. DETERMINANTS OF THE DISTRIBUTION OF NURSES IN PORTUGAL: DYNAMIC OLS MODEL

The so-called dynamic OLS application will be used to identify and quantify the determinants of the geographical distribution of nurses in Portugal over the 8-year period between 2002 and 2010[51] . In the econometric models applied - the same ones applied in the static analysis - the dependent variable will be the growth rate in the number of nurses per thousand inhabitants for the 8 years in question. Also for the variables included in each model to explain the distribution of nurses, their growth rate between 2002 and 2010 will be used. The estimated results for the dynamic models are shown below (Table 17).

Table 17

Results of the dynamic OLS models for the time interval between 2002 and 2010

Variables	Model 1	Model 2	Model 3	Model 4	Model 5	Model 6	Model 7
Medical	-	-	0,175 (0,214)	-	-	-	-
Population	12,126 ** (6,005)	9,287 *** (3,364)	-	6,980 ** (3,536)	-	8,866 *** (2,768)	8,084 *** (2,574)
Population_0-14	-7,242 * (3,681)	-7,202 *** (2,531)	-	-4,880 ** (2,152)	-	-6,424 *** (2,078)	-4,138 *** (1,444)
Tx_Mortality	0,775 (1,585)	-1,298 (1,034)	-	-	-0,625 (1,237)	-1,242 (0,947)	-
I_Aging	-2,183 * (1,211)	-1,831 ** (0,762)	-	-	-0,322 (0,767)	-1,634 ** (0,685)	-
I_Dependence	4,034 * (2,301)	4,054 ** (1,660)	-	-	0,926 (1,357)	3,211 ** (1,373)	-
MMasculinity	-8,906 * (4,823)	-5,137 (3,318)			-8,427 * (4,886)	-4,482 (3,139)	-3,286 (2,908)
Beds	-0,014	-0,024	-0,038				

51 It should again be noted that the distinction between static and dynamic models follows the distinction made by Correia & Veiga (2010) and may not conform to any other type of technical distinction between the two models.

	(0,092)	(0,057)	(0,089)				
I_Longevity	0,871	-1,432	-	-	0,552	-0,814	-
	(2,966)	(1,792)			(2,225)	(1,555)	
Nurse/doctor	-	0,721 ***	-	-	-	0,734 ***	0,724 ***
		(0,222)				(0,222)	(0,230)
IPC	4,924 **	2,961 ***	-	-	3,024 **	2,604 ***	1,635 **
	(2,095)	(1,114)			(1,396)	(0,920)	(0,734)
Hospital	-0,604 **	-0,302 *	-0,953 ***	-0,781 ***	-	-	-0,138
	(0,247)	(0,169)	(0,278)	(0,246)			(0,140)
Constant	-1,429	-0,943	1,935 ***	1,590 ***	-0,806	-0,830	-0,407
	(1,448)	(0,824)	(0,226)	(0,183)	(1,136)	(0,756)	(0,654)
Observations	251	253	251	306	306	306	306
Adjusted R2	0,094	0,606	0,015	0,039	0,065	0,6128	0,604
F-test	1,414	4,566 ***	4,084 ***	3,964 ***	1,214 *	5,038 ***	7,592 ***

Notes: Standard deviation values are shown in brackets; * indicates that the coefficient is statistically significant at a significance level of 10%; ** indicates that the coefficient is statistically significant at a significance level of 5% and *** means that the coefficient is statistically significant at a significance level of 5%.

Looking at the values in Table 17 for the dynamic model, we can see the low significance and low value of the adjusted value obtained in models 1 and 5, which shows that these are not the ideal models for analyzing the reasons behind the evolution of the distribution of nurses at municipal level in Portugal. Even so, it should be noted that for the remaining five estimated models, the F-test result is statistically significant at a significance level of 1%. It is worth noting the great weight in terms of explanatory power of the nurse to doctor ratio variable, as can be seen by the jump in the adjusted R^2 from model 1 to model 2. There is also an adjustment of around 60% in the models

2, 6 and 7, which means that the variation in the variables involved in each of the models explains around 60% of the variation in the number of nurses over that period of time. We should also note the low value of R^2 in model 3, which is surprising given that this model includes the variables number of doctors per thousand inhabitants, beds per thousand inhabitants and the presence of a central hospital. In addition to the low explanatory power, there was only individual statistical significance for the presence of a central hospital. For this *dummy* variable, it can be seen that the increase in the number of nurses seems to have an inverse relationship with the presence of central hospitals, which may mean that, although these are the places where nurses choose to work, they may be opting for other work contexts, probably motivated by the loss of services in these hospitals over this eight-year period.

There is also a weak explanatory power (low adjusted) of model 4, which is a model that includes the total population, the population aged 14 or under and the presence of a central hospital. This seems to indicate that the growth rate of these variables did little to explain the growth rate of the number of nurses between 2002 and 2010, despite the fact that the increase in total population and central hospitals was positively related to the increase in the number of nurses over the period (according to the results obtained for this model). The same is not true of the population aged 14 or under, whose growth rate seems to be negatively related to the growth rate of nurses per thousand inhabitants in Portuguese municipalities.

Model 6 has an adjusted value of around 61%, which means that the growth rates of all the variables included in the model explain around 61% of the growth rate in the number of nurses in Portuguese municipalities over the period considered (2002 to 2010) and with a confidence level of 99%. Looking at this model, we can say, with 99% confidence, that a 1% growth rate in the purchasing power of each municipality in this period implied a growth rate of around 2.6% in the number of nurses per thousand inhabitants. This result confirms the earlier trend that these professionals tend to move to places with greater purchasing power. There is also a positive relationship between the number of nurses per doctor and the number of nurses, which clearly suggests that nurses are more likely to work in places that can offer them greater autonomy as professionals. In other words, where there is a higher *skill mix* and, consequently, greater motivation for their work. Also noteworthy is the statistical significance obtained for the ageing index and dependency index variables in the same model. According to the results of the model, it can be said with 95% confidence that for every 1% increase in the ageing index in the Portuguese municipalities over the period considered, there was a reduction of around 1.6% in the number of nurses. In other words, this seems to imply a tendency for nurses to avoid the municipalities with the highest ageing indices (higher numbers of elderly people than young people), something that would not be expected at all (see Table 10). As far as the dependency ratio is concerned, every 1% increase in the dependency ratio in Portuguese municipalities over the 8 years under analysis corresponded to an increase in the number of nurses of around 3.2%. This value, which is high in model 6, is even higher in model 2 at the same significance level. In other words, there seems to have been an upward trend in the growth rate of the number of nurses in regions with more dependent people. This may be a reflection of the reform of the long-term care network that took place in the country over the same period, which implies a greater number of nurses treating this type of user. However, there seems to be a greater distance between these professionals and older people, who traditionally seek and need this type of professional the most.

It is also worth noting that model 6 shows a large weight in the growth rate of the total population and the population aged 14 or under. This statistically significant weight is, however, different in terms of its impact on the growth rate of the number of nurses. According to this model, every 1% increase in the population growth rate in a given municipality implies an increase in the number of nursing professionals in that municipality of 8.86%, which is quite significant. Conversely, if there is a 1% increase in the population aged 14 or under, there will be a percentage decrease in the number of nurses of around 6.42%. These factors seem to indicate that the number of nurses is growing in places where the total population is also growing and decreasing in areas where there is an increase in the young population, who, with the exception of the elderly, are the ones who most seek the care of these professionals.

Also noteworthy is the lack of individual statistical significance in the mortality rate variable in all the models in which it was tested, and it was not possible to draw conclusions either about the strength or the sign of the association, so future studies could look into this issue, which is considered to be of the utmost importance.

CONCLUSION

The aim of this research was to improve our understanding of the geographical distribution of the number of nurses in Portugal. It is believed that the results add value to the analysis of this issue by adding, to the traditional descriptive analysis of the data, the respective statistical contextualization with the other OECD countries and with the Portuguese reality itself. At the same time, empirical results have been added to the analysis of the problem of the distribution of the number of nurses in the Portuguese economy, making it possible to identify a set of factors that influence it. In this way, it is possible to offer a new perspective of analysis to all the political agents who make decisions in this field of health care provision. It is believed that new foundations have been laid for a more accurate assessment of the activity of nursing professionals over the last decade in Portuguese municipalities. These results could, for example, make it possible to ascertain whether or not new adjustment policies are needed in this area.

According to the statistics available for 2009, there were 5.6 nurses per thousand inhabitants, well below the OECD average of 8.5. It should be noted that, in 2010, the only Portuguese districts with a higher number of nurses per thousand inhabitants than the OECD average were Coimbra and Bragança. In absolute numbers, Lisbon and Porto were the districts with the highest number of nursing professionals in 2009. Even so, for the period from 2000 to 2009, Portugal was one of the countries with a higher average growth rate than its OECD counterparts, which means that Portugal has been making an effort to increase the number of these professionals. Also noteworthy for the same year is that the ratio of nurses to doctors in Portugal was 1.5, while the OECD average was 2.8. In other words, this figure represents a *skill mix* well below its OECD counterparts, which limits the autonomy of nursing professionals. In 2010, according to INE data, the average number of nurses per thousand inhabitants in Portugal was around 4, with some municipalities having no nurses at all and others having around 26 per thousand inhabitants, indicating clear asymmetries between the different Portuguese municipalities. In fact, calculating the Gini index made it possible to verify the existence of geographical asymmetries in the distribution of these professionals, despite evidence of a reduction in these asymmetries, since the value of the Gini index approached zero (0.505 in 2002 to 0.380 in 2010). In year-on-year terms, both the distribution of the number of doctors per municipality in Portugal and the purchasing power index showed signs of convergence, but to a much lesser extent than for nurses. The population moved in the opposite direction. The Gini coefficient increased from 0.604 in 2002 to 0.612 in 2010, confirming the worsening of regional asymmetries in terms of population distribution in Portugal in this period of recent history.

Using the econometric methodology that applies the least squares method, it was found that, in 2002, the main factors contributing to the increase in the number of nurses (per thousand inhabitants) at county level were: the number of beds per thousand inhabitants and the number of doctors per thousand inhabitants, something in line with what is mentioned in the literature in the area (Lin et al., 1997; Wong et al., 2009). However, the results also show the great influence of purchasing power on the retention of these professionals. This factor has a greater influence than the two variables mentioned above. Also noteworthy is the influence of the number of nurses per doctor, a possible *proxy* variable for the so-called *skill-mix* concept. The results obtained for this variable indicate that nurses also attach great importance to working in places where they are given greater autonomy. It should also be noted that this variable is related to the increase in the number of nurses over the last 10 years.

Applying the same methodology to 2010, in addition to seeing an increase in the explanatory power of all the models tested, we highlight the increase in explanatory power, compared to 2002, of the model with variables related to some of the population's health indicators (for example, the old-age dependency index and the ageing index). This result suggests a change in the distribution policies for nurses which, despite continuing to be strongly influenced by the presence of a central hospital, doctors and the number of beds per thousand inhabitants in 2010, also seems to be starting to be related to the health of the population covered - the number of nurses seems to be directly related to the ageing index and inversely related to the dependency index. This shows that in 2010 they were more present in work contexts with older populations, which may have contributed to a reduction in their old-age dependency ratio. This factor is further strengthened by the increase in the explanatory power of these demographic variables for the distribution of the number of nurses, since there was an increase in the adjusted coefficient of determination from 2002 to 2010.

The effect of the purchasing power index is surprising, in that it once again supersedes the effect of the number of doctors per thousand inhabitants, presenting itself as the variable with the greatest influence on the distribution of nurses at county level in 2010. The purchasing power of the population should not be overlooked when analyzing the distribution of the supply of some healthcare services, such as those associated with nursing.

As for the model that estimates the influence of the growth rate between 2002 and 2010 of the explanatory variables on the growth rate of the number of nurses distributed among Portuguese municipalities, there was a decrease in the explanatory importance of variables such as the number of beds and the number of doctors available per municipality. There has even been a decrease in their correlation. The growth rate of these variables has little explanatory power when it comes to the percentage change in the number of nurses per municipality between 2002 and 2010, which was not the case in the static models. In other words, although the presence of nurses may be related to these variables (static models), their variation in growth rates does not seem to be (dynamic model). Even so, the same model seems to indicate that nurses tend to grow in places where the total population is also growing, but to decrease in areas where there is an increase in the young population, which is surprising given that, with the exception of the elderly, these are the people who most need the care of these professionals.

With an opposite effect come variables related to demographic indicators of the population. There is a growing influence of these variables (population aging index and elderly dependency index) on the distribution of nursing professionals. The positive percentage change in the ageing index is negatively related to the increase in the number of nurses in the municipality, which seems to indicate a tendency for the number of nurses to move in the opposite direction to the ageing index. On the contrary, percentage increases in the old-age dependency ratio at county level lead to percentage increases in the number of nurses. In other words, there seems to have been a trend towards an increase in the number of nurses in regions with more dependent people between 2002 and 2010, probably reflecting the reform of the long-term care network that took place in the country during this period and which implied a greater number of nurses treating this type of older and more dependent users. In addition to the above, the purchasing power index reinforces its importance in explaining the variation in the distribution of nurses by municipality, suggesting that their distribution is clearly influenced by economic and well-being factors. Finally, the positive influence of the *skill mix* on the distribution of nurses by municipality should be noted, revealing that, in addition to the economic component, the professional autonomy component and work motivation are also factors that (albeit to a lesser extent) influence the increase in the number of nurses in the municipality.

In the future, it would be interesting to extend the time period of this study and specifically check the effects of the relocation of nursing professionals and their influence on reducing the mortality rate, since in this study no individual statistical significance was obtained for this item in the dynamic model. It would also be interesting in future studies to find out what factors motivate such large geographical differences in the ratio measuring the number of nurses per doctor, particularly between northern and southern European countries.

BIBLIOGRAPHICAL REFERENCES

High Commission for Health [ACS] (2011). Websig interactive platform. Retrieved on 26/11/2011 from: http://www.websig.acs.min-saude.pt./.

Aiken, L. H. & Cheung, R. (2008). Nurse workforce challenges in the United States: implications for Policy. *OECD Health Working Papers, 35,* OECD Publishing.

Alken, L.H., Clarke, S., Cheung, R., Sloane, D & Silber, J. (2003). Educational levels of hospital nurses and surgical patient mortality. *Journal of the American Medical Association*, 290, 1617-162.

Aiken, L.H., Clarke S., Cheung R., Sloane D., Sochalshky, J. & Silber J. (2002). Hospital nurse staffing and patient mortality, nurse burnout and job dissatisfaction. *American Medical Association, 288* (16), 1987-1993.

Antonazzo, E., Scott, A., Skatun, D. & Elliot, F.(2003). The labor market for nursing: A review of the labor supply literature. *Health Economics, 12,* 465-478.

Administraçâo Regional de Saùde do Algarve [ARS-AL] (2011). *Map of the composition of the ACES.* Retrieved11/12/2011from :http://www.arsalgarve.min-saude.pt/site/index.php?option=com_content&view=article&id=46&Itemid=59.

Administraçâo Regional de Saùde do Centro [ARS-C] (2011). *Map of the composition of the ACES.* Retrieved11/12/2011from :http://www.arscentro.min-saude.pt/ACES/Paginas/Aces3.aspx.

Baganha, M. I., Ribeiro, J. S., & Pires, S. (2002*).* The health sector in Portugal: how the system works and socio-professional characterization. *Oficina do CES n° 182*, Center for Social Studies, University of Coimbra.

Barros, P. P. (1999). Health policies in Portugal over the last 25 years. Retrieved on 15/10/2011 from http://momentoseconomicos.files.wordpress.com/2011/06/apesjan99.pdf.

Barros, P. P. (2009). *Health Economics - Concepts and Behavior.* Coimbra: Almedina

Barros, P. P. (2011). New user charges may push patients to go private. Diàrio Económico de13/12/2011 , 33-36. Retrieved on 15/01/2012 from : http://www.mynetpress.com/pdf/2011/dezembro/2011121329740b.pdf.

Barigozzi, F. & Turati, G.(2010). Human health care and selection effects. Understanding labor supply in the market for nursing. Retrieved 03/02/2012 from:

http://www2.dse.unibo.it/barigozz/nursesfinalhe24novemberpatrick.pdf

Baumann, A., Blythe, J., Kolotylo , C & Underwood, J. (2004). The International Nursing Labor Market. *The nursing sector study corporation*. Government of Canada. Retrieved 02/02/2012from :http://www.cna-aiic.ca/CNA/documents/pdf/publications/International_Nursing_Labour_Market_e.pdf

Bentes, M., Dias, C. M., Sakellarides, C. & Bankauskaite, V. (2004), Health care systems in transition: Portugal. WHO regional office for Europe on behalf of the European Observatory on Health Systems and Policies. Copenhagen.

Birch, S., O'Brien-Palas, L., Alksnis, C., Murphy, G. & Thompson, D. (2003). Beyond Demographic Change in Human Resources Planning. Center for health economics research and evaluation. University of technology of Sydney

Blegen, A. M., Goode, C. J. & Reed, L. (1998). Nurse staffing and patient outcomes. *Nursing Research*, 47 (1), 43-50.

Bloor, K. & Maynard, A. (2003). Planning Human resources in health care: Towards an economic approach. An international comparative review. *Canadian Health Services Research Foundation*. University of York. Ottawa. Retrieved on 04/02/2012 from : http://www.chsrf.ca/Migrated/PDF/ResearchReports/CommissionedResearch/bloor_report.pdf

Branco, A. G. & Ramos, V. (2001). Primary Health Care in Portugal. *Revista de saùblica, 2*, 5-12.

Berlinier, H. S., Ginzberg, E.(2002). Why this hospital nursing shortage is different? , *American Medical Association*, 288 (21), 2742-2744.

Bigbee, J. (2008). Relationships between nurse- and physician-to-population ratios and state health rankings. *Public Health Nursing*, 25 (3), 244-252.

Briggs, B., King, L., Basu, S., Stuckler, D. (2010). Is wealthier always healthier? The impact of national income level, inequality, and poverty on public health in Latin America. *Social Science & Medicine, 71* (2), 266-273.

Buchan, J. (2002). Global nursing shortages, *British medical Journal,* 324, 751-752.

Buchan, J. & Calman, L. (2005). Skill-Mix and policy change in the health workforce: Nurses in advanced roles, *OECD Health Working Papers,* 17, OECD Publishing.

Budge, C., Carryer, J. & Wood, S., (2003), Health correlates of autonomy, control and professional relationships in the nursing work environment. *Journal of advanced nursing,* 42 (3), 260268

Bureau of Health Profession [BHP] (2002). Projected Supply, demand and shortage of registered nurses: 2000-2020, The national center for health workforce analysis, Government of the United States of America . Retrieved 10/15/2011 from :

http://www.ahcancal.org/research_data/staffing/Documents/Registered_Nurse_Supply_Demand.pdf

Carr-Hill, R. & Jenkins-Clarke, S. (2003). Improving the effectiveness of the nursing workforce. *Center for Health Economics working paper, 44,* University of York.

Carrie, V., Harvey, G. West, E. Mckenna, H. & Keeney, S. (2005). Relationship between quality of care, staffing levels, skill mix and nurse autonomy: literature review. *Journal of Advanced Nursing*, 51 (1), 73-82.

Ciutan, M. & Chirac, N. (2009), The territorial distribution and use of emergency hospitals in Romania. *Health Management,* 1, 67-72.

Comissão nacional de desenvolvimento da cirurgia de ambulatrio [CNADCA] (2009). Outpatient surgery in Portugal: state of play. Retrieved on 12/04/2012 from : http://portal.arsnorte.min-saude.pt/portal/page/portal/ARSNorte/Conte%C3%BAdos/Not%C3%ADcias/CNADCA_Julho2009.pdf.

Conselho de Enfermagem [CE] da Ordem dos Enfermeiros (2003). Competencies of a General Care Nurse [Electronic version]. *Revista Divulgar*, 7-24.

Correia, I. & Veiga, P. (2010). Geographic distribution of physicians in Portugal. *Journal of Health Economics,* 11, 383-393.

Cottrell, A. & Lucchetti, P. J. (2012). Gretl User's Guide - Gnu regression, econometrics and TimeSeries Library Retrieved on 12/04/2012 from: http://sourceforge.net/projects/gretl/files/manual/

Davidson, R. & MacKinnon, J. G. (2003). Econometric Theory and Methods. Oxford University Press.

Decree-Law No. 305/81 of November 12 (1981). Provisions on the approval of the nursing career. Official Gazette, Series I, 2998-3004.

Decree-Law No. 104/98 of 21 of April (1998). Provisions on the creation of the Order of the nurses and their respective statutes. Official Gazette, Series I-A, 1739-1757.

Decree-Law no. 353/99 of September 3 (1999). Establishes the general rules governing the teaching of nursing in higher polytechnic education. Diário da República, Series I-A, 6198-6201.

Decree-Law No. 413/71 of September 27 (1971). Promulgates the Organization of the Ministry of Health and Assistance. Official Gazette, Series I, 1406-1434.

Decree-Law No. 414/71 of September 27 (1971). Establishes the legal regime that will allow the structuring and functioning of the various differentiated groups of employees of the Ministry of Health and Assistance. Official Gazette, Series I, 1434-1445.

Decree-Law no. 161/96 of September 4 (1996). Approves the regulation of nursing practice in Portugal. Official Gazette, Series I-A, 2959-2962.

Decree-Law no. 437/91 of November 8 (1991). Provisions on the approval of the legal regime for the nursing career. Official Gazette, Series I-A, 5723-5741.

Decree-Law No. 122/2010 of November 11. Establishes the number of remunerative positions in the categories of the special nursing career. Diário da Repùblica, Series I, 50995101.

Delamaire, M. & Lafortune, G. (2010). Nurses in advanced roles: A description and evaluation of experiences in 12 developed countries. *OECD Health Working Papers*, 54, OECD

Publishing.

Direcçâo Geral do Ensino Superior [DGES] (2012). indice de cursos do ensino superior em 2012. Recuperadoe m1 6/06/2012d e:

http://www.dges.mctes.pt/DGES/pt/Estudantes/Acesso/Genericos/IndicedeCursos/

Directorate-General for Health [DGS] (2011). National health programs. Retrieved on 19/11/2011 from : http://www.dgs.pt/default.aspx?cn=60766101AAAAAAAAAAAAAAAA

Doherty, C. & Hope, W. (2000). Shared governance - nurses making a difference. *Journal of Nursing Management*, 8, 77-81.

Donahue, M. P. (1996). *Nursing, the finest art- An illustrated history*. Mosby-yearbook

Elliot, S., Fisher, J., Wennberg, T., Stukel, J., Skinner, S. & Sharp, J. (2000). Associations among hospital capacity, utilization and mortality in US. *Health Services Research*, 34 (6), 13511362.

Nursing School of Coimbra [ESENFC] (2011). Postgraduate study plan. retrieved12/11/2011from :

http://www.esenfc.pt/esenfc/ensinos/index.php?target=showContent&id=100019&ano_lectivo=&tab=pe

Finlayson B., Dixon J., Meadow S. & Blair G. (2002). Mind the gap: the extent of the NHS nursing shortage. *British Medical Journal*, 325, 538-541.

França, H. H. (1987). The Burnout Syndrome. *Revista Brasileira de Medicina*, 44 (8), 197-199.

Friesen, D. (1996). Skill mix literature review. *Healthcare Management*, 9 (2), 48-52.

Gavin, M. & Wakefield, S. (1999). Shared governance: time to consider the cons as well as the pros. *Journal of Nursing Management*, 7, 193-200.

Gibbs, I., Mccaughan, D. & Grifiths, M. (1991). Skill mix in nursing: a selective view of the literature. *Journal of Advanced Nursing*, 16 (2), 242-249.

Graça, L., Henriques, A. I. (2000). Evoluçâo da Pràtica e do Ensino da Enfermagem em Portugal. Texts on health and work. Retrieved on 04/01/2012 from: http://www.ensp.unl.pt/lgraca/textos62.html

Gujarati, D. N. (2004). *Basic Econometrics* (4th Edition). McGraw-Hill.

Heyes, A., (2005). The economics of vocation or why is a badly paid nurse a good nurse? *Journal of Health Economics, 24*, 561-569.

Henwood, T., Eley, R., Parker, D., Tuckett, A. & Hegney, D. (2009). Regional differences among employed nurses: a Queensland study. *The Australia Journal of Rural Health*, 17, 201-207.

Hess, B. (1994). Shared governance: innovation or imitation. *Nursing Economics, 12* (1), 28-34.

National Statistics Institute [INE] (2011). Statistical database of Portugal. Recuperadoem13/10/2011de

http://www.ine.pt/xportal/xmain?xpid=INE&xpgid=ine_indicadores&indOcorrCod=0000890& context=bd&selTab=tab2

Janiszewski, G. *(*2003*)*. The Nursing Shortage in the United States: an integrative review of the literature. *Journal of Advanced Nursing,* 43*, 335-350.*

Law no. 111/2009 of September 16th. Amends the statutes of the Portuguese Bar

Association.

Nurses. Official Gazette, Series I, 6528-6550.

Law no. 56/79 of September 15 (1979). Provisions on the formation of the National Health Service. Official Gazette, Series I, 2357-2363.

Lin, G., Burns, P. A. & Nochajsky, T. H. (1997). The geographic distribution of nurse practitioners in the United States. *Applied Geographic Studies*, *1* (4), 287-301.

Manton, L., Corder, L., & Stallard, E. (1997). Chronic disability trends in eldery United States population: 1982-1994. *Proceedings of the National Academy of Sciences of the United States*, 94 (6), 2593-2598.

Marques, C. B. (2006). Skill mix - Sharing functions makes intervention capacity more profitable. *Jornal do Médico de Familia*, 1 (12), 54.

Martinez, L., F., & Ferreira, A. I. (2010). *Data analysis with SPSS - First steps*. Lisbon: Escolar editora.

Matias, A. (1995). The health care market. *Working document n⁰ .5⁄95*. Publications of the Portuguese Association of Health Economics.

Maynard, A. (2006). Medical workforce planning: Some forecasting challenges. *The Australian Economic review*, 39 (3), 323-329.

Mendes, F., R., Mantovani, M.,F. (2010). Current dynamics of nursing in Portugal: A

representation of nurses. *Revista Brasileira de Enfermagem,* 63 (2), 209-215.

Mckeown, M. (1994), Skill mix reviews: the need to be aware. *Nursing Standard*, *8* (32), 37-39.

Meadows S., Levenson, R., & Baeza, J. (2000). The last straw - Explaining the NHS nursing shortage. *King's Fund*, London.

Munga, M. A. & Maestad O. (2009). Measuring inequalities in the distribution of health workers: the case of Tanzania. *Human Resources for Health*, 7 (4), 1-12.

Needleman, J., Buerhaus, P., Matke, S., Stewart, M.& Zelevinsky, K. (2002). Nurse-staffing levels and the quality of care in hospitals. *New England Journal of Medicine,* 346 (22), 17151722.

Nightingale, F. (1860). Notes on nursing- what it is, what it is not. *D. Appleton Company,* New York. Retrieved on 16/11/2011from :

http://digital.library.upenn.edu/women/nightingale/nursing/nursing.html

Nogueira, M (1990). *History of nursing*. Porto: Ediçôes Salesianas.

Nunes, L. (2003). *A look at the shoulder, Nursing in Portugal (1881-1998)*. Loures: Lusociência.

OECD/European Union (2010). Health at a Glance: Europe 2010. OECD Publishing.

OECD/European Union (2011a). Health Statistics database, retrieved from the internet on 01/11/2011

OECD/European Union (2011b). Health at a Glance: Europe 2011. *OECD Working paper, OECD Publishing*.

OECD/European Union (2011c). OECD Stat Extract - Gross Domestic Product per head, *OECD Working paper, OECD Publishing*.

OECD/European Union (2011d). Divided we stand: Why inequality keeps rising. OECD Working paper, *OECD publishing.*

Ordem dos enfermeiros [OE] (2011a). Nursing in Portugal. OE publications,

recuperadoe m1 5/11/2011d e:

http://www.ordemenfermeiros.pt/publicacoes/Documents/Brochura_10anos2008.pdf

Ordem dos enfermeiros [OE] (2011b), A Profissâo, Retrieved on 02/11/2011 from : http://www.ordemenfermeiros.pt/AEnfermagem/Paginas/AProfissao.aspx

Ordem dos enfermeiros [OE] (2011c). Regulaçâo do Exercicio Profissional do Enfermeiro-Decreto-Lei n.° 161/96, de 4 de Setembro (Com as alterações introduzidas pelo Decreto-lei n° 104/98 de 21 de Abril), retrieved on 20/10/2011 from : http://www.ordemenfermeiros.ptlegislacaoDocumentsLegislacaoEnfermagemREPE.pt

Ordem dos enfermeiros [OE] (2011d). Important legislation on nursing. Retrieved 11/11/2011from :

http://www.ordemenfermeiros.pt/legislacao/Paginas/LegislacaoEnfermagem.aspx

Ordem dos enfermeiros [OE] (2011e). Nursing Career - Relative consultation. Retrieved on 15/11/2011from .

http://www.ssm.gov.mo/design/news/Document/p_CarreiradeEnfermagem-ConsultaRelativo.pdf

Ordem dos enfermeiros [OE] (2011f). Statistical data 2000-2010.Retrieved on 13/102011

from
http://www.ordemenfermeiros.pt/membros/Documents/OE%20Dados%20Estat%C3%ADst
i cos%20-%202000-2010.pdf

Portal da Saùde (2011). The History of the SNS. Retrieved 23/11/2011 from : http://www.minsaude.pt/portal/conteudos/a+saude+em+portugal/servico+nacional+de+saude/historia+do+sns/historiadosns.htm

Ministerial Order no. 239/94, of April 16 (1994). Disposiçâo sobre a regulamentaçâo dos cursos de estudos superiores especializados na área de enfermagem. Official Gazette, Series I-B, 1821-1825.

Porter O'Grady T. (1992). *Implementing shared governance: creating a professional organization*. St Louis, MO: Mosby

Pronovost, P.J., Dang, D., Dorman, T., Lipsett, P.A., Garrett, E., Jenckes, M. & Bass, E.B. (2001). Intensive Care Unit Nurse Staffing and the Risk for Complications after Abdominal Aortic Surgery. *Effective Clinical Practice*, 4, 199-206.

Quintas, C., Farto, J., Rosa, M., & Santos, M. (2007). History of nursing in the 1980s [Electronic version]. *Revista Percursos,* Special issue of Nurses' Day. Retrieved on 10/11/2010 from: http://web.ess.ips.pt/Percursos/pdfs/per_esp_dia_enf.pdf

Rosado, A., Rolo, A., Silva, A. & Castel-Branco, C. (2007). Nursing in Portugal: from the end of the eight hundred to the middle of the nine hundred [Electronic version]. *Revista Percursos,* Special edition of Nurses' Day. Retrieved on 10/11/2010 from: http://web.ess.ips.pt/Percursos/pdfs/per_esp_dia_enf.pdf

Ricardo, D. (1965). *Principles of political economy and taxation*. Lisbon: Calouste Gulbenkian Foundation.

Richardson, J. (1997). How much should we spend on health services. Center for health program evaluation, Working paper, 63.

Reinhardt, U. E. (2003). Does the aging of population really drive the demand for health care?, *Health Affairs*, 22 (6), 27-39.

Robinson, V. (1946). White caps - The history of nursing. *Journal of Medical Association*, 135 (2), 129.

Segre, M. & Ferraz , F. C. (1997). The concept of health. *Revista de Saùde Pùblica*, *31* (5), 538542.

Simoens, S., Villeneuve, M. & Hurst, J. (2005). Tackling nurse shortages in OECD countries. OECD Health Working Papers, 19, OECD Publishing.

Skillman, S., Palazzo, L., Keepnews, D., & Hart, L. (2005). Characteristics of registered nurses in rural vs. urban areas: implications for strategies to alleviate nursing shortages in the United States. Center for Health Workforce Studies, Working Paper, 91, University of Washington.

Taylor, L. J. (2007). Optimal wages in the market for nurses: An analysis based on Heye's model. *Journal of Health Economics*, 26 (5), 1027-1030.

Tierney, A.J. (2003). What's the scoop on the nursing shortage? *Journal of Advanced Nursing,* 43 (4), 325-326.

Toyabe, S. (2009). Trend in geographic distribution of physicians in Japan. *International Journal for Equity in Health,* 8 (5).

Wade, G. H. (1999). Professional nurse autonomy: Concept analysis and application to nurse education. *Journal of advanced nursing,* 30 (2), 310-318.

Webster's New World Medical Dictionary - Third edition (2008). New Jersey: Wiley Publishing

WHO/World Health Organization (2011). Definition of heathcare. Retrieved on 17/12/2011 from : https://apps.who.int/aboutwho/en/definition.html

Williams, A.(1978). *Need - an Economic exegenis.* Economic aspects of Health services. London: Martins Robertson

Wong, S. T., Watson, D. E. & Young, E. (2009). Supply and distribution of primary healthcare registered nurses in British Columbia. *Healthcare Policy, 5* , 91-104.

Zurn P., Dal Poz, M., Stilwell, B. & Adams, O. (2002). Imbalances in the health workforce. World Health Organization, *Briefing paper*, Geneva.

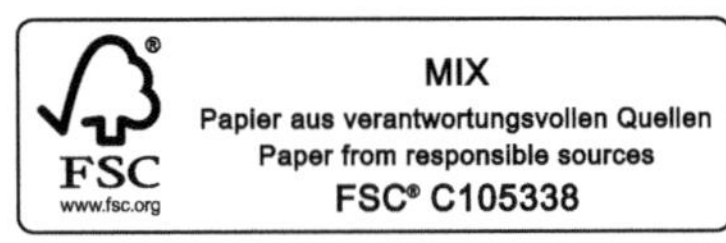

Printed by Books on Demand GmbH, Norderstedt / Germany